The Amazing Life & Journey of a Natural Childbirth Doctor

Victor M. Berman, MD

By James Hathaway, AAHCC

Marjie & Jay Hathaway, AAHCC

Victor M. Berman, MD AAHCC

This book is birthed through the many meetings, locations, and time it took to formulate the content with the subject. It is done with the consent and direct input of said subject. Vic Berman has read this book and wholeheartedly endorses it!

This book contains general information, ideas, etc. Please check with your own health care provider(s) and use your own good judgement in order to determine what information applies to your specific situation and which ideas and information are appropriate for you. Every situation is different. We make no guarantees or assurances of any kind to anyone. Only you can make the important decisions you will face during pregnancy, labor, and birth. The information in this book is presented in the hope that it will inspire you to seek the best and safest options for you, your baby, and your family.

The Bradley Method® and American Academy of Husband-Coached Childbirth® are registered Trademarks with the U.S. Patent Office.

AAHCC

Academy Publications, Box 5224, Sherman Oaks, CA 91413

ISBN:0-931560-05-5

The Amazing Life and Journey of a <u>Natural Childbirth Doctor</u>
Victor M. Berman, MD

We are proud to call Victor Michael Berman M.D. a friend, family and colleague who has inspired us and given us great inspiration and opportunity to learn from a truly gifted doctor.

Like all of us, Vic didn't start out as a doctor... Or did he? Well of course not but maybe he always had the inspiration of becoming one. We are going to look at this extraordinary life and learn many things that will help future generations come into this world in a much better way.

So, before we go any further. We want to give a great BIG thanks to Vic and his departed wife Salee Berman, CNM who have helped us on our journey of expanding The

Bradley Method® of Natural Childbirth throughout the world.

Dedication

To all the babies yet to be born... we acknowledge how many have taken incredible steps and been on journeys to ensure that this process will always be available to you and your families.

This book was written to honor Dr. Victor Berman and his wife, Salee, for their dedication to the pregnant woman and her unborn baby. It is our hopes that this book will help women have a better birth and learn that they have choices and that the natural process is amazing and that every woman should not only be encouraged, but supported in having a natural birth. It's not only best for baby... but also mom, dad, and their growing family!

We believe that it is from the forging of alliances with The Bradley Method®, Marjie, Jay & James Hathaway, Dr Robert Bradley, Dr Thomas Brewer, Marian Tompson (La Leche League), Our patients, and the countless Bradley educators that NACHIS, the term Birth Center, and Natural Childbirth are not only possible, but thrived and continue to thrive throughout the world.

Don't Mess with Mother Nature!

Find a BradleyBirth.com teacher today!!!

Table of Contents

From the Beginning

Victor Michael Berman was born at the Brooklyn Jewish Hospital on February 8th, 1931 in Brooklyn, New York.

His father used to talk about how Vic was the result of a partial Cesarean. It wasn't until he was in medical school that he realized that they probably gave his mother an extreme episiotomy, which they referred to as a partial Cesarean.

His father was also warned that Vic might never see, due to the fact that he had a cut near his eye and was probably delivered with forceps. Perhaps this laid the framework to his devotion to making every birth a truly Happy one.

Father and Mother

Vic's father, Abram "Abe" Berman, was an immigrant who was born in 1900 and made the journey from Pinsk, Russia to the U.S. as a baby. He eventually met and married Vic's mother Dinah, "Diana", who was born in New York in 1898. Vic was their first and only child for 12 years.

Vic's father's family made the pilgrimage to the United States because of the anti-Semitism (hostility to or prejudice against Jews) growing in Russia & Europe. They immigrated legally, when Abe was only 2 years old, to the land of Freedom and Opportunities! What an incredibly brave and noble trek to undertake, so that their legacies would have the very best chances in life.

Abe sold women's clothing in the city, until he found his true calling of creating lodges or getaways! Diana was a schoolteacher during the school year, but ran the lodges with her husband, Abe, during the summer months.

Abe passed away at age 62 of complications to kidney issues. Diana fared better and passed away at the age of 90 in 1988. For the grandchildren they got to enjoy, they were known as "Grandpa" & "Grandma".

As far as the family legacies (children) were concerned, their grandparents were American and Abe & Diana spoke only English to them.

Diana's family were also from the same community in Russia, as Vic's Father's family. Both sides of Vic's family made this epic pilgrimage to the new world. Her 5 siblings, two brothers and three sisters were all born on the Uncasville farm in Connecticut.

Diana was the first woman in their family to go to college and was a schoolteacher, as well as being a wife, mother, and eventually entrepreneur of their new adventure together.

Stability

A child typically grows up in a stable environment where they live year-round. For Vic, this was not the case. He would live in the country during the summer months and would go back into Manhattan, Greenwich village, to a new apartment and area during the fall and winter each year as he was growing up.

His grandparent's farm was the closest to a consistent home that he would know for the first nine years of his life.

Grandparents

Both sets of Grandparents and their families came to America in the hopes of living the American dream and starting a new life of limitless possibilities for not only them-selves, but especially for their legacies (children) to come far after they had expired from this earth.

Upon entry into the U.S. it was very common for travelers to modify their family names as to fit in better to their new country's style. This was very true with Vic's ancestors on his mother's side who came with their surname of "Lifschitz and modified to Lifschutz, a small change, but one they had hoped would lessen ridicule with their neighbors.

Vic's mothers' parents were Abram & Bashi. Apparently, Abram was a common name amongst the members of their village or area in Russia.

Chance of a Lifetime

How Vic's Grandparents wound up not only living in Uncasville, but obtaining a 100 acre farm. It was a life altering opportunity... seemed it was more of a gift/opportunity than a loan.

A Count, who was trying desperately to solve the "anti-Semitic" situation came up with a plan to expand the Jewish population and footprint by loaning money and property opportunities to Jews seeking a new and better life.

At a party, this Count was talking with Vic's grandfather, Abram and offered him a farm in Uncasville, Connecticut. Abram looked at the Count and simply responded, "Vy Not!!!".

This simple exchange would transform Vic's family legacy and ultimately the experiences he would be part of as he grew and expanded his own horizons.

Uncasville farm grew to much more than just a farm, it was a safe haven and eventually the start of many businesses over the years.

Family Farm, The Uncasville Farm

Vic's grandparents had a wonderful farm in Uncasville, Connecticut. 100 acres, brimming with cows, chickens, and an assortment of other animals, from mules to cats to round out the workload. They grew corn, green beans, peas, cabbage, cucumbers, lettuce, etc. I'm sure seasonal rotations occurred as well.

Chickens for meat and eggs, Cows for milk, cheese, etc. This was a wonderful place to visit, eat from, and experience nature in all her glory. This would be a source of stability for Vic as he grew up as a child. Literally the only stable environment he knew. His parents would change their home in the city each year with the start and completion of the school year. During the summers they would head back to the family farm, after vacating their apartment in the city.

This was just their routine. Vic's mother was a Schoolteacher and his father sold women's clothing, but during the summer months they would head up North, back to their proverbial roots and expand on a getaway that would eventually rise to become a summer resort, which could accommodate 100 guests.

After nearly a decade, Vic's parents branched out to another location and left the Uncas lodge in the capable hands of Vic's Uncle, who turned it into a children's summer camp.

"Wow, That's Some Baby!"

On the Uncasville farm, Bashi (Vic's grandmother) had 4-6 cats roaming the house at all times and 5-20 cats outside which were semi-wild.

One day we were in the house and one of the cats, who was a large kitten and daughter of a house cat, was in need of some attention. My cousin picked her up... and all exclaimed, "be careful... it's a baby!" My cousin said, "Wow, that's some baby!"

"Some Baby" became this precious kitten's name. Even when she became a grown-up cat, the name, "Some Baby", remained.

Lemons into LEMONADE!!!

Although living in Manhattan during the school year, Vic's parents would go out to the countryside to visit and escape the hot city summers on his mother's parents farm.

This was a time when air conditioning wasn't readily available, and people had to seek out ways of staying cool during the summer heat. One of these ways was to get out of the city and go into the country where it was cooler and there were other things to do.

Vic's parents and their friends had made reservations at a hotel to get out of the city and where it was cooler. A week before their trip was to begin, they got a call from the hotel and were informed that their reservations were cancelled and that they were not welcome. This was a heaping load of lemons... instead of wallowing in their sorrows... they turned it all into LEMONADE!!!

Abe and Diana purchased some used circus tents, one for men and one for the women to have separate sleeping quarters. This gave their friends a place for them to join them out at their family farm and escape parts of the hot and humid summer months. This was way before Woodstock!

This took off and Vic's father Abe had a new trade and job opportunity. He was in women's retail sales and now was the manager and proprietor of this new venture. This first site became The Uncas Lodge in Uncasville, Connecticut in 1930; with a main Lodge and eventually 20 cabins. This would be the site of Vic's upbringing and exposure to nature and all her glory, during his first ten years of life.

There was a kitchen and dining hall with a large area for people to congregate. With individual cabins for families and couples to come and just enjoy the hospitality and country life. This exposed Vic to a variety of experiences and the opportunity to meet new and interesting people.

This taught Vic many, many, different lessons. First how to interact with people. Second how to entertain them. Third what hard work could accomplish. Fourth that nature is wondrous and there is much to learn from her. It was a bountiful life with incredible adventures to be had.

His parents were extremely hard-working and were great examples for Vic to learn from. His father wound up building and maintaining many of the dwellings that they established at their resorts. Over the years they wound up creating and then selling many different locations.

Legacies (Other Lodges)

Although the Uncas Lodge was growing in popularity. With success, comes strife. Vic's father looked for a new location, being that the lodge they had started, was not on their own land, but that of Diana's folks.

Many more Summer Vacation Resorts would be created, grown, and eventually sold to make way for their next adventures and locations.

Vic learned much through the ups and downs his parents endured during their creation, growth, expansion of the many properties they cultivated into successes. It took a lot of hard work and dedication... values that taught Vic well.

Uncas Lodge, 1930.

Camp Colebrook, Colebrook River, Connecticut (Formally a Country Club.) 1939.

Pine Crest, West Cornwall, Connecticut 1942.

Echo Lake Lodge, Vermont 1943.

Pine Crest, West Cornwall, Connecticut 1946. (second time around... they purchased it back from the owner who did not make a good go of it!)

Birdland, Central Valley, New York. Formally an estate. 1948.

Starting from just used circus tents and grew to cottages and communal gathering and eating areas. With music, laughter, and great camaraderie. Summer fun and relief at its Best!

A simple get-away turned out to be quite the adventure and a lucrative one at that.

Lodges/ Resorts

The **Uncas Lodge** had its humble beginnings simply as used circus tents that had been erected to help give refuge from the brutal summers in Manhattan. Eventually they would be transformed into a main house along with 20 individual cabins for guests to reside in.

Before Vic was even born or perhaps being part of the legacy... Vic's parents trans-formed the tents to cabins in 1930. Vic himself was born February 8th, 1931. Apparently, Uncas Lodge was not the only thing created that summer!

For approximately a decade, Uncas Lodge rose up and became a fixture in Connecticut. Eventually Vic's uncle took over the location and used it for a children's camp until it was sold.

1939 brought about a change and the creation of **Camp Colebrook** in Colebrook River, Connecticut. Originally a country club with 10 buildings with 3-7 rooms each. There was a chicken coop that also stored hundreds of hunting & fishing magazines that Vic spent countless hours reading.

Pine Crest was created in 1942 in West Cornwall, Connecticut. With a Main house and 8 small cabins. A couples retreat, primarily. 20-40 year olds. One of Vic's jobs was to keep the kerosene filled for the water heaters on each cabin, daily.

Echo Lake Lodge   Brandon, Vermont 1943 (possibly Plymouth region now). 20 cabins, lake adjacent. There were waterfront and wooded view cabins, common hall, dining and dancing area.

Pine Crest (again) 1946
After selling Pine Crest in 1943, they acquired it again. The new owners weren't able to make a go of it, so Vic's parents bought it back.

Birdland 1948 Central Valley, New York, Once owned by a very famous family, was a Lodge building, little pond. Housed around 80 people. To this day... no one knows why the name. Of course, there were birds in the area, just like all the other lodges.

Over more than a decade they would create, modify, upgrade, and sell or buy a resort. Many incredible times, friendships and laughter were had by all.

Description of the Lodges/Resorts

Turning onto a country road, you would make your way to a Lodge. Parking was first come first serve. There were people around dressed very casually. In fact, the staff were usually in t-shirts and shorts. Vic's father referred to their resorts as, "Camps for Adults!" These were get-a-away retreats that were, for the most part no frills no fuss. Just a place to escape the hustle and bustle and even more importantly, the extreme heat of the summer.

Walking into the lodge there was a reception area where you would be greeted and told which cabin you would be staying in. Keys were a formality that most never even used. This was a safe place and there weren't others around, except for staff and the other guests.

You would proceed to your cabin. It was a separate cottage with a shared bathroom between two separated rooms. Or a cabin with its own bathroom. Some rooms with fireplaces. $50, $60, or $70 a week, including all your meals.

Singing, acting, ping pong, boating, swimming, hiking, bird watching, nature loving, exploring, biking, dance hall with live music. A three-piece group resided there the whole summer.

Food: spaghetti, chicken, beef, bacon and eggs, baked goods, pies, fresh fruit, & turkey every Sunday. Tables in the dining room.

No internet, no phones in the cabins, no tv, no sirens, honking, no traffic.
Clean air. The night sky was something magical. In the city you could hardly tell that a star even existed, but at the lodge, you could look up and feel and see a blanket of stars that covered the sky. It was a slice of heaven.

Besides the guests, we had a myriad of visitors. Everything from frogs, to squirrels, to deer, raccoons, cats, and dogs, birds, skunks, butterflies, grasshoppers, fish, fireflies, etc.

Special Occasions: Memorial day, (Decoration day), 4th of July, & Labor Day.

Campfires at night... in the open field. Sit around the fire and tell jokes and sing-alongs. Marshmallows were a staple item.

Surroundings, all green and lush, a break in the forest. Closest towns between 9-11 miles away.

Bonded Together!

Every young child should grow up with a dog! For Vic, this was Pal, a black and white Border Collie. Although Pal was actually Vic's grandparents' dog who resided with them on their farm... didn't stop the summers from being theirs together. Pal was a beloved friend and playmate. Pal only knew Yiddish, because Vic's grandparents only spoke to Pal in Yiddish.

Although there was a language barrier between Vic & Pal, it never caused them a moment's hesitation to be life-long buddies and watch out for each other. Pal was the ideal playmate and protector. They would spend the summers together, getting into mischief whenever they could. They were inseparable.

Being a border collie, Pal also enjoyed the water and they would spend time in, on, and out of the water. Whether it be boating, swimming, hiking, or taking the occasional nap together. Their adventures were vast, and this strengthened Vic's love for animals and nature and set the groundwork for many dogs, especially to be in Vic's life.

Prayer

There is a prayer that sums up what it feels like to have a dog in one's life. ***"God, make me as wonderful as my dog thinks that I am!"*** Powerful words, but anyone who is fortunate enough to have a life companion from one of these furry critters knows what we are talking about. It is truly remarkable to have the unconditional love that a pet brings to your life.

Companions

Vic had many companions through the years. Starting with Pal and the latest was Katie, an English Bull Dog. Mookie, Gaspar, were earlier companions.

Vic and Salee knew how special and important a dog is to one's family. When they heard that the Hathaway's had a loss in their family, with the passing of their dog Duchess, they went out and found a wonderful addition, but not a replacement for their beloved dog.

Ilio, which is Hawaiian for dog, was a golden retriever & pit bull mix. She was a golden-haired beauty and was a tremendous part of The Hathaway's growing family.

Country Style Fishing and Fun

We would go down to the lake, a small pond my grandfather made by making a dam in a small brook that ran through the woods. It was large enough to float a few rowboats and had a wonderful population of small fish including sunfish and yellow perch.

How to dig for worms...
Chicken yard-worms are attracted to chicken waste, have to "fight" the chickens for choice worms! Put worms in tin can with a little dirt to cover them to keep them moist.

Fishing pole
Tall (at least twice my height) about 2 meters. Thickness (three child fingers in diameter) around the size of a quarter.

Trim off stick of all small protruding branches and leaves.

Tie a string to small end of narrowing pole (fishing line, if available).

Tie float (2-3 inches of dry wood) onto fishing line. Total length of line, same length as pole or a bit longer.

Small fishhook tied at end of line (we used real fishhooks! Not bent pins as some would describe).

How to fish from shore
Choose a likely looking spot, preferably one with partial shade and a place to sit!
-Near sunken logs or overhanging trees, near Lily pad's or "sea weeds"
Put worms carefully on hook.
Toss line out... And keep an eye on the float!
When the float moves or jiggles a bit, a fish is nibbling on your bait!
When the float dives down and swims away... then you know the fish has been hooked!

Pull your rod up and you may have a nice fat sun fish or maybe a yellow perch! These fish, although small are excellent eating, but watch out for the bones!!!

Pal

Pal and Vic would get into mischief, but they always shared in the fun. A relationship which sparked Vic's love for dogs and having many over the course of time.

Vic fell in love with English bull dogs, which began with Gaspar... then Mookie, who was used as a therapy dog and even visited Salee in the recovery room, which made a world of difference. Katie was Vic's latest English Bull Dog.

Dogs are an incredible addition to one's family and become icons in this environment. A life is only half lived without one's best friends.

Vic's Perspective

Although he belonged to my Grandparents in the winter... during the summer he was mine or more likely, I was his. A Border Collie named Pal, we were inseparable. We used to hike in the woods and explore mother nature together. He helped expand my world and gave me the opportunities to see nature in all her glory.

This dog was fluent in the Yiddish language, my grandparents only spoke to him in their native language. But when I came to visit... he had to learn my native language of English. This taught an incredible lesson that I utilize even to this day! Although you may speak one way... to interact with others, you must learn even a basic form of communication. As a doctor it is was hard to get this through to my colleagues, but I knew that you had to find common ground to be able to communicate well. I always took time to understand my patients and to make sure that they also understood me... Our common ground tool was The Bradley Method.

I learned many things from Pal; Patience, persistence, caring, trust, obedience, loyalty, etc.

Farm life was an incredible place to experience nature at her best!

ANIMALS

On his grandparent's farm there were a plethora of animals to observe, play, and learn from.

Cats

Indoor cats (4-5) and outdoor cats (20 or more)... by and large I was the only one able to get near the outside cats and eventually pet them. Their kittens were my first exposure to another animal raising their young. I remember seeing these new lives nursing away and enjoying being in a loving environment. We had a small black kitten that we named Peter... who turned out to be a girl and was renamed to Petra!

Cows

I learned to milk cows. And learned first-hand that in nature it is always better directly from the source... whether milk or fruit or produce, etc.

I can remember my cousin visiting us on the farm and having fresh milk for the first time. If you don't know by now, fresh milk and that watery substance you purchase at the store are not that same at all. My 6-year-old cousin Suzanne took a big drink of the cow's milk... and proceeded to spit it out! Crying and saying, "I don't like cow's milk... I like real milk out of the bottle!"

My grandfather sold his milk to a local dairy. He would store this milk in the barn/ building. A trough ran river water around the large "silver" containers of stored milk, keeping it fresh until it was sold and picked up. Remember, this was before refrigeration and people had ice boxes which were replenished with ice frequently.

I observed the necessity of having mother and child together. The cows nursed their baby calves, cats & dogs did likewise.

One experience was to stick my finger inside a calf's mouth and have them such on my finger in such a strange way... almost like sandpaper, yet softer and bigger protrusions. These calves can really suck! Pop!

No tractor, just two work horses on the farm. We were warned as children to never get behind the horses, because they could kick you and kill you. I chose to steer clear of their backsides!

I remember the man who came to shoe the horses. On a red-hot fire, he would prepare these metal U shapes that would eventually become their Horseshoes. He would hammer them into place, and I was amazed to see him bend the horses back leg between his own legs and hammer this object onto the horse's hoofs... this was indeed a very powerful professional. Once again, an incredible lesson... observing the talents of someone who was an expert and literally knew how to avoid being a casualty of one's profession!

Chickens

Eggs... a golden nugget of nutrition and my introduction to the reproductive process. Chicken yards were a great resource for worms... and I liked to go fishing. Once I turned over the soil outside of the coops... it literally was a race between me and the chickens to catch the Best worms! And I would put them in my little can and rush down to the lake to possibly catch supper. ...the early bird catches the worm, and with it a nice dinner!

Boating

Once my mother got a call from a woman frantic that I was in the middle of the lake, jumping out of a boat and swimming around... all by himself! My mother calmly said, "It's all right, he knows how to do it!" ...I was only 7 at the time. I was one with the water and eventually fell in love with the sea.

Canoes

In the summer, my job was to keep the boats & canoes clean and remove any water. They were a wonderful way to get exercise while on the water and basking in all of nature's glory.

Sailing

We used to take a rowboat and place a small concrete block inside of it. Then stick a pole inside the block and attach a sheet to the pole and it would catch the wind and wind up sailing across the lake... what a thrill! Downside was I had to row all the way back because it was a small lake and you can't fight the wind.

[This was a gateway experience which increased Vic's passion to the point of becoming a Captain* and sailing from California... through the Panama Canal and making it to Florida. Note: He also sailed in

Hawaii, Virgin Islands, Bahamas, England, Mexico, Catalina, San Francisco Bay, Hudson River... to name a few locations]

*U.S. Coast Guard Licensed Captain

Tonsils

Vic was around 4 years old and his mother told him that they were going on an outing to the Zoo. They got into the car and headed down the road, but wound up at a huge building and was admitted into the hospital.

On the operating table and a heavy accented man tells Vic to count backwards, "now count after me, 10... 9... 8... 7... 6... woke to a lot of pain in his throat and he tells us that there is no amount of ice cream that could ever make up for this. Stayed in the hospital for a few days and then went home. Smell of ether and thinking about this disturbs him, even to this day.

They used to say that a good anesthesiaologist likes the smell of ether.

Stability & Little Red School House

When Vic was 9 his family finally settled down, at least during the winters in Manhattan, New York. This afforded Vic with a more stable environment and brought him to the *Little Red School House*, which would help educate and even introduced him to his future wife, Shelly.

Youth

During his younger years, Vic changed elementary schools, many times, and found it all very confusing.

When he was 9, they finally settled in Greenwich village so he could be closer to school and finally had a more stable life.

Little Red School House

Little Red School House, a private school featuring progressive education, a new way of looking at life and thinking. Many of the ways of thinking and approaching problems would help Vic all his life, even in medical school.

At the Little Red School House, you were a person and not just a member of the flock... a sheep! This was a progressive school and those who attended, usually graduated from college.

Unfortunately, Vic did not complete is schooling at the Little Red School House. The lodges/resorts made them move around, but his experiences have stayed with him and have forever made an indelible mark on him.

The school may also be responsible for his children, since this was the catalyst in meeting future wife.

My High School Sweetheart

The Little Red School House where Vic attended elementary school was where he would meet his future wife, Shelly. They knew of each other, but it wasn't until their High School years that they became an item. Their romance blossomed. For a time, they had a long-distance romance.

More to come, later in the book!

Parents Flexibility

Vic's mother was a schoolteacher and his father was a salesman of women's clothing in the city. This gave them the ability to migrate in the summers to the countryside.

His mother was a full-time teacher, but when Vic was around 10 changed to a substitute teacher. This enabled her to leave the school year early and go help set-up the lodge before the summer rush.

His father was a jack of all trades and actually maintained and built many of the structures they used.

Life Lessons... City vs Country Life

As Vic was growing up, life taught him many lessons living in the city during the year and especially the time he got while also living in the summers in the countryside. Both venues brought different and unique challenges that he would learn and grow from... some more challenging than others.

Bee stings

I was walking along, at the age of 7-8, and kicked at a hole in the ground which sent debris into it... Then a swarm of bees emerged, with a lot of buzzing and I quickly ran away. Later I came back and kicked even more debris and again a bigger swarm came out and I ran away. The third time... I did the same thing and turned to run, but tripped and fell and was attacked especially on my leg. I Stumbled home and was bedridden for what seemed like weeks. The lesson was... don't pick on someone smaller than you, especially if they have friends, are faster, and armed with pointed objects to do harm!

Vic's Father became highly allergic to bees. Vic had just gotten his license and had to rush his father to the hospital, which did save his father's life.

How to treat a bee sting
Baking soda was the remedy. You would put a pinch on the wound and add water.

As a child, a doctor would make a house call to treat Vic. Their bedside manners made him feel that, it was the duty of a great doctor to make a patient feel better and understood.

In medical training... Each professor or instructor/doctor had their own way of interacting with the patient or not.

His Trouble with Gas...

Their resort was a good size and had a kitchen with at least four stoves in it. Vic was fond of nature and had started a butterfly collection. To preserve his specimens, he would use the gas from a stove to sedate and eventually preserve his growing collection. As long as he didn't light the burner, he could use the gas to preserve his butterfly.

Lessons come in many forms... And this one will never leave him. He prepped the butterfly by putting it into a glass jar and holding the jar over the burner without a flame. It wasn't too long before it happened... KA BOOM!!! An explosion ensued and it singed his eyebrows, yet fortunately everything else was fine. Turned out that although he had carefully extinguished the pilot light on one of the stoves... an adjacent stove's pilot light was still lit! He was incredibly lucky to have not gotten seriously hurt during this explosive event! KA BOOM!!!

There is Another...

Having had an adventurous youth, an event was soon to change his life... forever.

Vic was now 12 years old and having been the only child, he was informed that their Triad was about to have another. I don't believe that Vic fully grasped, at that moment, how this event was to forever change their lives and expand their hearts... in very good ways.

Well the day came, and Vic was informed that he was now, The BIG Brother!" But when would he meet this new addition to their family? As a youth or for that matter... anyone waiting to meet a new addition to the family simply can't wait for this meeting to occur.

Vic recalls this introduction to their family. Usually this simply was a new building or location for their

Summer resorts. But this time there was a special twist to this new surprise.

As a youth, he was restricted from visiting in the hospital... not permitted to see his newly born sister. This maybe where Vic was introduced to the notion that often, you must think outside of the box... or miss many of the wonderful experiences and surprises life has to offer.

His father had scoped out the hospital and discovered that there was a way for Vic to get entrance into the maternity ward without going through the main door. For you see... children were restricted form going into the maternity ward... ironic? (Children not allowed!)

He and his father went to the back of the hospital where there was door that opened to a staircase that led upstairs to the nursery observation window with chicken wire running throughout the glass. Here they both were able to get to see, Greta Berman swaddled in a blanket and sleeping in her bassinet. Vic fell in love with his baby sister and they remain very close today.

This experience changed his life and thinking and gave him pause to the miraculous event of a new life's effect on one's world. This possibly planted the notion that families should never miss these precious, life-altering events and experiences... "Life changers!"

This event changed the way he would live his life and realized that sometimes you have to think outside the box... instead of living in it!

Shoot for the Stars
(Dad telling sister... not nurse, but doctor!)

When my sister told my father that she wanted to be a nurse when she grew up... he kindly said no and that she should become a doctor. No limits for my family. This instilled in me the notion to shoot for the stars and not accept limits that I might set for myself.

This helped me throughout my life and gave me the chance to soar... so I followed his advice and indeed became a doctor... and so did my sister Greta Berman. She has a PhD in art history from Columbia University, NY and later became an instructor at the Juilliard School in Manhattan, NY. She is still teaching there. Greta and her husband travel the world giving lectures.

Changing Schools

Although residing in Manhattan during his younger years, Vic's family did move around, and he attended different schools while his family set up new locations for their summer retreats.

School kids can be mean, and Vic took his share from confrontations at schools that were supposed to teach him and keep him safe... a few broken lips and bruised eyes did occur. Many of those were lessons and he benefitted from the experiences by developing a tougher shell, but still keeping a side of him as the protector. This served the thousands of women and families that walked through their doors once he got their Practice & Birth Center, NACHIS, up and running.

His childhood gave him an extreme love for Nature and to experience the different sides she has to offer. Learning from the woods and forest to the jungle of Manhattan to eventually finding a love for the sea and becoming a true captain of many vessels and even sailing from Los Angeles all the way down South America to the Panama Canal and making their way to Florida where he and Salee retired for some years.

They had a lovely custom-built home on Little Gaspar Island, FL. Vic designed their home and had an architect finalize the plans.

Unfortunately, their beloved home was too far away for friends and family to visit easily... so they ultimately decided to move back to Southern California to be closer to all.

Schooling

Attended public schools, up to three different ones a year, due to demands of the lodges opening and closing schedule.

Moved to Manhattan, NY at 9 years old to 45 Morton St., Greenwich Village, New York.

Attended _Little Red School House_.

At 12 went to a <u>public school _PS3_</u>.

At 13 went to a private school <u>City and Country School</u>.

At 14 went to first year (first semester only) of high school in a town called Central Valley in New York State and attended _<u>Central Valley High School.</u>_

Only Jew in the school... beaten pretty severely. Came home, mother screamed, "What Happened to You".

Parents went to principal and he told them that, "that could never have happened at his school!"

Stuyvestant for remainder of High School – renowned school.

Vic wanted to go to the science school, *Stuyvestant,* (fathers' Alma Mater), or Bronx Science... because they have girls! Won't take a student in middle of the year so go to *Stuyvestant* to start. Passed exam for *Bronx School of Science* and *Stuyvestant*. Wound up staying through high school. It was a hard school and taught him something (taking test, a lot of technical information of chemistry, biology, physics). Did not like the strict atmosphere Was not a good student. Moved back to Greenwich village (Manhattan) during high school. 30 min commute for mother to get to work.

Because of moving around... resentful of taking tests. Mother taught me to read very early pre-kindergarten. In 7th grade mother called in because he couldn't read... he could read better than the teacher!

Father worked from home in real estate.

All through high school he had major mis-understanding of the system and answering examination questions. Treated well and not well. Was a bit rebellious of the system... problem changed my whole thinking and interaction with the world. Didn't like the system of working for grades. Understanding was more important than taking a test to prove a process and not rewarding in the knowledge itself.

One of the Cool Kids

The school bell had wrung, and a mad dash was made out of the school and onto the steps leading in or out of school, as the case may be.

I was standing next to a good friend who had already fired up one of his leashes... you know, one of those items you can't live without and in due time will take your life.

He took a drag and seem to be content with the toxic gases permeating his lungs and giving him a euphoric feeling and sensations of relief.

But in his haste, he had forgotten a book he needed to take home, so he proceeded to hand off this lit stick of death and happiness. "Here, hold this for me, I forgot my history book!"

There I was, holding a lit cigarette so I said to myself, "Let's take a puff and see what's all the fuss about?

Having the opportunity, I proceeded to raise this longed for token of insanity to my lips and proceeded to take a drag, puff, oh whatever you call it... THIS WAS DISGUSTING!!!

It tasted awful and hurt my lungs as I coughed and wheezed this elixir of death and desire.

In short, this was my one - and only - time taking part of this absolutely disgusting habit! One of my finer decisions in life!
If only those who started and never begun... life is sweeter when you don't have a leash keeping you hostage to a glowing stick of disaster and incredible cost and destruction!

My advice... never get on this road... its literally a dead end.

Change of Seasons

Vic's mother Diana was a schoolteacher and would make the trip from Manhattan to Brooklyn each school day on the subway, which was a half an hour to over an hour commute each day (depending on traffic and timing of the train).

She did this for nearly a decade until her attention was needed more at the resort.

She would need to leave the school semester early to be able to help opening the lodges before the start of summer.

So, they made the decision to have her change from being a full-time teacher to a substitute teacher who had the flexibility to change her schedule and hours. Besides, the resort was really their passion and was the primary source of stability for their family.

The Kindness of Strangers

Vic's first year of High School at Central Valley, New York. His parents had decided to keep their resort open through Christmas time.

It was the middle of winter and Vic was somewhere around 14-16 years of age. He had not learned to drive yet, not even driving his Grandfather's regular car.

It was very cold out and snow on the ground. His Father woke Vic at some ridiculous hour 5-6 am in the morning. His car was stuck in the snow and he needed Vic to come and help him get his car unstuck.

As they were out there on a country road, near their home, a local country doctor drives up and offers to help. Vic was impressed that he would stop and give aid, in a non-medical way. A cheerful fella who had finished a House Call and was more than willing to lend a hand.

Many people are cranky and hard to deal with when they wake... Vic remembers thinking that he too was good at waking up and being cheerful and felt that he too could make a good doctor. Also felt that he was good at getting along with new acquaintances. This was in part due to interacting with hundreds of new people each and every summer.

He met hundreds of people every season. And the first or primary objective was to make them feel welcome as if they were still at home. And it occurred to Vic that this kind of interaction could be very useful as a doctor.

Vic was turned off by the attitude of many doctors who had an attitude that he was annoying them or taking up their time, but the country doctor gave Vic pause, and gave him perspective, that to be a good doctor, you needed to interact with your patient on a human level and always be respectful and take the time to be not only a caregiver, but a friend.

Side note:

Vic is delighted that his granddaughter has also become a doctor. She has followed in his doctoring footsteps and those of her father, who is also a doctor. Her mother is also a doctor. She continued the tradition of attending Howard University Medical School in Washington, DC.

The Entertainer

Growing up in a summer lodge exposed Vic, not only to nature, but to the arts as well. This helped instill a passion of all things artistic. He was a singer, musician, comic, and whatever else was needed around the lodge. This gave Vic a greater understanding of the needs and communication levels required when interacting with others... great skills that would be good to use as an Obstetrician.

Vic's mother was also an accomplished artist. Working in the medium of paint, she had incredible talent and apparently passed this along to both her son & daughter.

Vic works in the mediums of, paint, clay, wood, stone carving, renewals, cloth, etc.

Music or Medicine

It is not known by many, but Vic is a very talented musician and folk singer. Way back in his young adult years, he contemplated being a Professional Folk Singer... he would entertain the guests at many of the family lodges and he was very good and talented at this.

His grandmother gave him a guitar and he loved this gift and mastered it.

One day walking down the streets of Manhattan he stumbled on a discarded Civil War era banjo. He saved it from the trash truck coming down the street and took it with him. It was nice, but in poor condition. Parts were broken, and it was not able to be played. Stuck in the back of his closet and going from location to location as he grew up, it still traveled from home to home for decades.

Eventually Vic had a patient whose husband was a guitar maker and ask if he could repair this instrument in lieu of partial payment for his services. Vic was glad to make this deal in the hopes of bringing this magical musical instrument back to life.

Upon the return of this instrument he was informed that this was a very special instrument and had great value.

Little did Vic know that in the hard times he had a treasure hidden away and eventually was brought back to life and bringing music to this world once again. Vic's sister, Greta is in possession of this treasure today!

Go Out West Young Man

During the Summer of 1948 I ran into a gentleman at my parent's vacation resort. He recommends that I go out west to college... because of the different perspective on life.

This stayed with me and probably gave me a path that lead me out there.

A simple 10-minute talk influenced me. Also, met a couple who had a birth in South America and their enthusiasm was intoxicating and probably motivated me to learn more about childbirth.

Colorado Living

The University of Colorado, nestled at the base of the Rocky Mountains was to be home for Vic during the next four years of his college education.

Denver is a unique city. Touted as being the "Mile High City", which it is... but it's nearly flat as a pancake. As you fly from California to Denver, you literally fly over an incredible mountain range that is beautiful and awe inspiring. Once past the Rockies you head east over flat terrain to make it to a very unique airport. It reminds me of Circus Tents, but they are the airport terminals shrouded in a sea of white tarps or canopies, which were designed to mimic the Snow-covered Rocky Mountains, themselves. Boulder is literally on the outskirts of Denver, easily seen from each other.

Boulder... Denver... Colorado... has much to offer. Nature is all around you, along with all the luxuries of a modern city. Vic took full advantage of his surroundings and even joined a hiking club and scaled several mountain ranges during his time there.

One can only imagine being a Biology student and having nature in all her glory, merely steps away... or at least a short drive.

This experience was a wonderful, life changing journey, which opened doors to new people and experiences that taught him many lessons. Nature is not meant to be explored only in a book... just like in Vermont, he enjoyed communing with nature and learning all about the Science of Biology. This helped to fulfill a part of an empty void he was missing, but later in life, again he would need to learn and grow even more.

Sharing Nature & Their Lives

Vic was at the University of Colorado, while Shelly was studying in Ohio.

After spending only vacations together, Vic and his *Little Red School House* Sweetheart decided to make it official.

During the Winter Break of Vic's senior year. Vic and Shelly decided to get married, back in Manhattan.

Vic's father Abe, being in the textile business, and being approximately the same size as Vic, was able to acquire Vic's suit for the wedding ceremony, without him being there.

After their wedding, Vic and Shelly headed back to the University of Colorado, where Vic achieved his Bachelor of Science Degree in Biology. Shelly also achieved her Bachelor of Arts Degree in Teaching (Education).

They had an apartment together in Colorado and once they graduated, headed back to Manhattan, New York, to be near family and friends.

Vic & Shelly were both schoolteachers… along with both their mothers. Shelly had a job at a Junior High School and Vic and his mother & mother-in-law were all teachers at the same elementary school.

Teachers Blood

Vic's mother was a teacher in Brooklyn and made the commute from Manhattan to Brooklyn every school day. No wonder he also sought out this career and became a biology instructor.

Although he achieved his family's legacy of being a teacher, he felt there was something more for him.

So, after being a teacher for four years he went back to school and eventually became an M.D. Eventually he specialized in Obstetrics.

Greta also followed in their mothers' footsteps and is still teaching at the Julliard School in Manhattan, New York.

In-between Years

Vic was licensed with the New York City Board of Educators. New York State vs New York City... this was not transferrable.

Before pursuing his medical education, Vic contemplated combining his love of science with his talent and passion for art. He thought of being a medical illustrator.

Assistant

Vic discovered a position for a "Laboratory Assistant," at a New York City High School, but was really teaching the class. This did not require a teaching certificate to be doing this, or did it? Anyway, it gave Vic a great opportunity to teach, learn, and explore science and realize that he wanted to do more. He did this while completing the required teaching certificate needed for him to be the primary instructor. He got credit for on the job experience and achieved a regular teaching license in General Science for Jr High School, instead of a substitute teacher license. This afforded him the ability to also teach in Elementary schools as well.

He taught elementary school for 2 years. General Science in Jr High School for an additional 2 years.

First Pregnancy

After his wife Shelly gave birth to their first son, Ira, Vic decided to go to medical school to become a doctor. His decision was influenced by the experience they had during their pregnancy. They both read Dr. Grantly Dick-Reads book, *"Childbirth Without Fear"*.

This book had inspired them, but something was lacking. They both felt that they longed for answers and training on how to give birth. His book explained ideas of childbirth, but did not prepare you for the birth at all.

During their pregnancy they had to go from Manhattan to Connecticut and back down again. They were instructed by their doctor to not drive and that a train would be much better and safer for a pregnant woman. So… Vic & Shelly drove to the train station and Vic put Shelly on the train. Vic then traveled by car, following the train to Connecticut. In retrospect this seems ridiculous. Why would a train be better than their own car? This is one of those moments that shapes your understanding and need to do things better, and not necessarily as one is told. Commonsense needs to be a factor as well.

Back home they waited for the eventual birth of their child. Probably the greatest suggestion they got during their pregnancy was from an older doctor that suggested that they stay home as long as they could before going to the hospital, as birthing takes a long time and they would just be waiting at the hospital instead. Apparently, Shelly was doing a great job and waited longer than anticipated... until they felt it was time to leave for the hospital. Vic recalls how his car was wedged in between two other cars and took some maneuvering to finally get on the road to the hospital.

They finally arrived at the hospital and Vic took Shelly into admitting and got her situated.

He was not permitted to attend the birth and at that time, fathers were basically sent home to wait for a call to come and retrieve or meet their new family. But Shelly was much further along in the process. They asked Vic to stay and wait for the results... soon he was informed that they had a son... now he was excused to go home!

Mother and baby were to be kept for several days until permitted to leave the hospital and make the journey home.

A Path Unknown

Vic always had a desire to do more, be more, but how? He had his bachelor's degree in Science and was teaching junior high kids, but something still stirred deep inside him. He always had a love for art and wondered if he could do something to combine the two? So, he thought of being an illustrator for medical books, but that didn't pan out.

He tried being a researcher, but that too did not pan out. He finally stumbled into a position as a laboratory assistant, but this was really a teaching position. It did not require a teaching certificate, and all he had to do was take an additional class. He got credit for on the job experience instead of continuing with a sub license. Now he could get a regular teacher license, which made it possible for him to teach in Jr High School. He taught elementary school for 2 years. General Science in Jr High School for 2 years.

Although teaching students was rewarding, he still desired to do more. But what? Vic applied to many Universities trying to get into medical school. His father thought the world of his children and when Vic's sister Greta told their father that she was thinking of being a nurse, with a gleam in his eye said nicely, "No… Doctor!" He migrated to the U.S from Pinsk, Russia and knew that his children could do anything they set their minds to do. Greta got her doctorate in Art History and is still teaching at Julliard in Manhattan.

Advisor

So how could Vic accomplish his burning desire to be a doctor when he got such a late start to do this?
One session with an Academic Advisor changed his path. Sitting down, this session simply asked some questions and by the time their meeting was over, Vic was on a mission to become a doctor.

Howard University

This was a monumental task and how was he going to be able to start medical school having started later in his life? At first, he applied to the usual suspects, but was not accepted. He even applied to medical schools outside of the U.S. and was accepted into a program in Italy, but then he also got accepted into Howard University in Washington, DC. Not in their medical program directly, but in Pharmacology.

Backdoor
A two-year program that he had heard could also be used as a backdoor access into medical school... which it was. During Vic's first year he applied to the medical program at Howard and was accepted. Finishing his first year he went on to finish the four-year medical program as well. Vic and Shelly got an apartment in Silver Spring, Maryland, for the 5 years, 1 in pharmacology, and 4 in medical school.

He did his rotations, but always had a connection or passion for Obstetrics. While at Howard he saw and was part of countless of births. The potential for learning and experiencing births was tremendous.

This was when Vic got to see the difference between a drugged/medical birth and a natural/emergency birth. The medicated births he attended and helped or saw the administration of drugs and anesthesia was eye opening. Especially in comparison to the last-minute walk-in who literally gave birth in the emergency entrance.

Forever Changed Him

During his Senior year in medical school, while observing at DC General Hospital, a woman came into the ER and right in front of him had her baby! Just squatted down and a baby was now in her hands... no drugs, or being shaved, no epidural or IV's, no interventions at all!! Just a healthy baby and a confused mother and staff. Perhaps this was one of the moments to forever change Vic and give him the foundation and knowledge that nature does indeed know what she is doing and that doctors are there for emergencies and not to create them!

Mother and baby were great and were whisked away into a room to perform additional procedures on the two of them.

Normal "natural" birth could be calm or frantic and the moms seemed to experience more/less pain, their babies were beautiful, healthy and alert... and did not suffer from life-long effects and damage from their exposure to drugs. Unlike the medicated babies who literally had to be brought back from the brink of death due to the procedures they had to endure.

There was a difference... **BIG DIFFERENCE!!!**

A baby being brought into this world without drugs versus a baby being exposed to drugs was like the difference between night and day! Vic realized that what he and the hospital were doing was putting those babies at risk and was absolutely the wrong thing to be doing. They had been telling these moms that if it hadn't been for them and the procedures done that their babies would have died. Vic knew and saw how it was actually the opposite, and it was their skills of bringing a baby back that was the miracle. They literally were putting both mom and baby at risk and causing the medical emergencies they were trained for. They were thanked for saving lives, but in reality, they had been putting lives in danger.

[Occasionally, a woman would come into the hospital, literally at the last moment, and have their babies in the entrance to the hospital. The babies were born pink, alert, and full of life, unlike the babies that were being born upstairs in the delivery rooms. This was a revelation! A seemingly meaning-less event and new understanding would change Vic's course and give him a cause and reason for what he would dedicate his life too.]

Knowing the Difference

Now Vic had a problem... he knew the difference! And little wheels started spinning as he progressed with his training and experiences. But this birth will be forever etched in his mind and knowing that not all births need to be interfered with.

Vic's Perspective (Teaching)

My first day on the labor & delivery floor. I learned a lesson, unintentionally, that stayed with me the rest of my career.

I entered a large room with several women in labor. In one corner there was a young woman screaming hysterically with each of her contractions, as if she was sure that she was going to die! No one had taken the time to explain to her the normal progression of labor.

Though she was very loud, no one was paying any attention to her. I was wearing a white coat (but not yet a doctor, just a student), and I went over to her and asked, "what was the matter?" (between contractions), screaming loudly she exclaimed, "these contractions are killing me! Am I going to die?"

*I tried to console her and to try and ease her pain...
without the "standard of care" another dose of
medications.*

*I simply talked with her... explained how contractions
do not last forever and that nature was giving her rest
periods. She was surprised by what I was telling her.
She thought that this was simply going to continue
until her insides ruptured and the baby would gush out
onto the floor.*

*We worked together through the contractions and she
learned quickly how to relax in the rest times and work
with and not against her body during a heavy
contraction. There is a beginning and end to each
contraction and your body will adjust accordingly
during the whole process.*

*It is amazing to see the difference between a woman
who works with her body, letting the contractions do
their jobs, opening parts of her body in preparation for
the eminent birth itself. Rather than listening to
screams and torture of a woman who does not know
what is happening to her and is scared to death,
literally. Bradley training helps women have joyous
birthing experiences, versus painful, drugged, horrific,*

hospital births I participated in during my medical training... it is what we are taught! Protocols, she was unmarried or unpartnered.

This amazing event transformed Vic into something much greater than being a doctor. In this moment he expanded his role as healer to also being a teacher and advocate to the unborn. This scared woman didn't know what was happening to her and Vic took the time to explain what was happening. He told her how her contractions have a rhythm and that they do not last forever. That a contraction starts and lasts for about a minute and then is subsided and nature then gives you a break. This made all the difference in the world!

Now this teachable moment made it possible to help this young woman get through her labor and eventual birth of her baby in a kinder and gentler manner which helped avoid un-necessary interventions and drugs.

She was very grateful, both for the explanation and help, but also for the attention that I, "a doctor" (in her eyes only... I was still just a student wearing a white coat!)

This experience taught me two important lessons: 1. Attention from a doctor is extremely important! 2. How important it is for the patient to understand what is happening to them, I later learned how important childbirth classes would be.

Kind words can and do change the world! Sometimes we simply need to know what is to be asked of us which in turn makes it possible to reach our goals. Just imagine how women today need a teacher/ doctor who takes the time to explain the process instead of denying the magic moments of pregnancy and birth.

Vic was well-known for taking the time, always saying positive aspects of a labor and birth, not just being a lifesaver, but rather a saver of the natural process.

Trust Me I'm a Doctor!
Vic has an extreme talent for making a person belief whatever he tells them. He would look at a wall and emphatically tell you that there were 1346 bricks that made up the wall... and you would trust him... why wouldn't you? This is an incredible skill and help with patients to calm them down. Knowing something without a doubt is very reassuring.

Ethics in His Family

Honesty was a guiding principal of their lives. Vic's parents were great role models of hardworking, honest people.

Training and the Medical Approach

Dr. DeLee is touted as the father of modern Obstetrics, Rubbish!

DeLee's formula for medical birth management:

1. *Universal sedation of women.*

2. *Universal episiotomy.*

3. *Universal forceps extraction of fetus.*

"So frequent are these bad effects that I have often wondered whether Nature did not deliberately intend women should be used up in the process of reproduction, in a manner analogous to that of salmon, which dies after spawning." Delee

In part utilizing Delee's formula, standards were mandated for the training of doctors. To be a good doctor, every women coming to a hospital must be separated from their loved ones, be stripped of their clothes, get an I.V., be shaved, vaginal exams, strapped down for delivery, administer drugs, have the baby removed from their mother with forceps, baby be confined to the nursery.

These procedures, as standards, are barbaric and outrageous to routinely expose all women & their babies to.

So-Called Modern Approach
Especially during the 20th century, many procedures were mandated on women during labor and delivery. These were never implemented for the laboring women, but rather for the comfort and access of the doctor and facility.

1. **Separation** from loved ones... never done for the woman, but rather a way to control the environment for staff.
2. **Stripped** of clothing and dignity.

3. A woman was restricted to **lie on her back** during labor and/or delivery. This was done so the doctor could observe the vagina in a less awkward way.

4. **Shaving** was done to reduce the doctor's & hospitals exposure to fleas and lice. Not done for delivery reasons. Not needed for the majority of women in the first place.

5. The **I.V.** was a way to restrict a woman's movement and, in essence, chaining them to their beds. Also a gateway to drugs & procedures.

6. **Restriction of food and drink**. Dr. Curtis Mendelson made this a standard back in the 1950's. Because of a drug, scopolamine, women were put into a psychotic state where they would thrash around potentially causing damage to themselves and those around them. During delivery the woman would be strapped down in leather restraints and their head immobilized. Some drugs would cause nausea and if she vomited, she could inhale and choke on her own vomit and possibly die.

7. **Fetal monitoring** brings with it a host of risks.

8. **Ultrasound** Still this day has not been proven safe!

9. The use of **Drugs**. Whatever and wherever the mother's body is exposed to any drug, will eventually get to the baby... there is no such thing as a completely closed system, when it comes to the human body.
10. **Stirrups** prevented natural & efficient (for the mother) positioning during the Birth.
11. **Episiotomy** It was the job of the obstetrician to make sure that every woman received an episiotomy, whether she needed one or not!
12. **Forceps** used during medicated births due to the restrictions. Mothers body no longer able to work with her contractions. Forceps Increased the likelihood of bleeding and possible damage to the head and skull of the baby.
13. **Cesareans** are a great tool and resource, but should only be done in an emergency situation, which is far less than 10% of the time. How is it possible that the Cesarean rate is over 30%?
14. **Nursery** care. Babies require attention, love, and support. Separating a mother from her baby is barbaric!

Curtis Mendelson, obstetrician and cardiologist wrote an article in 1946 titled, "The aspiration of stomach contents into the lungs during obstetric anesthesia" which was published in the American Journal of Obstetrics and Gynecology. Coined as Mendelson's Syndrome. Today the answer to this problem isn't to restrict food or drink, but to NOT strap the head down and if the patient vomits, to tilt or turn the head to evacuate the content. Commonsense approach to a rare problem... (restrict all for the very few... craziness)

Game Changer by Two

Background: in order to understand the story, some background is necessary.

I was a third-year medical student. This was the first time a student actually lays hands on a live patient. The class is divided into small groups, so that they can be given personal attention and supervision.

When I was in training, it was before the invention of ultrasound for diagnostics in pregnancy. Twins were frequently surprise discoveries at their births.

Careful examination including auscultation, "listening", it was possible to discover twins... occasionally!

With this in mind, the significance of the following story will be better appreciated.

One day when I was in a group that had not yet examined "real" patients... I met a classmate who was in a group that was examining obstetric ("pregnant") patients.

As he met me in the hall, he said, "I just had a wonderful experience, I heard the heartbeats of twins!" He was excited and asked me to join him and listen to the Twins!

We went into the room and found a young woman in bed and asked her if I could listen. She happily agreed (she had only discovered that she was carrying twins a short while ago). With A stethoscope I begin to listen... I was thrilled to hear two separate and distinct heartbeats, both in the normal range rate for a term pregnancy this is approximately 140 beats a minute. Somehow this experience of feeling the positions and hearing the heartbeats affected me in such a way that I immediately felt that I wanted to be part of the process of taking care of pregnant women and helping them to have their babies.

It was a rather short experience... But it changed my whole life! I have maintained my interest in obstetrics, *but became interested in many other fields as I experienced them.*

My Son David

Born at New York infirmary for women and children. Manhattan, New York.

Shelly stayed with her folks during the last few weeks of the pregnancy. Vic had to stay in Silver Springs, MD while he was completing a semester at Howard University.

Unfortunately, Vic was taking his Finals when David emerged into this world. Finishing one final, Vic got on a bus and made his way to his growing family and to meet David for the very first time. He then had to get back on the bus make his way back to his next Final Exam.

David followed in Vic's footsteps by also becoming a doctor, as well. Also, he is an Alumni of Howard University. David is a very Renowned and Prestigious Pediatrician in Torrance, California. Head of Pediatrics at Torrance Memorial Hospital.

Vic is very proud of David and wanted us to document this within the confines of this book.

Let Me Control You... You Will be My Hands!

During his fourth year of medical school in 1963, Vic was given the opportunity to deliver his first baby. Being a newbie and not knowing what or how to do it... of course he had learned the basics and had taken the tests, but now it was real... no net! He was ultimately the one in charge. Fortunately for Vic a wonderful nurse was assigned to him and was there to guide him through the entire process... not verbally, but to actually guide him through the process.

When it was time to deliver the baby, she got behind Vic and put her hands just short of his hands on his arms and used herself as kind of an external skeleton manipulating him and guiding him to aid in the delivery of the baby. This was a thrilling experience, almost like being outside of one's body and observing the whole experience yet performing all the tasks at hand. This gave him great confidence and knowledge of the typical process and he was glad to have such an amazing teacher to get him through his first hands on experience.

Chickens with Their Heads Cut-off

Being part of a medical rotation process is a little like going through a year with your head cut-off... You scurry frantically trying to find a fit or place that you love to continue to learn and become a specialist at.

Rotations were an opportunity for the students to get a taste of the different areas of medicine and a foundation for General Practice (GP's), while possibly helping guide a doctor to focus on the one that they were most passionate about. There was Internal Medicine, Psychiatry, Emergency Room, Surgery, Pediatrics, Family Medicine... and of course Vic's favorite area, Obstetrics!

He says the thrill of seeing a new life come into the world is truly one of the greatest experiences a person can have. He further believes that it is a shame for any couple to miss these magical moments and how medicated births rob the entire family of these miracles. Also, they are not best for baby! They may relieve pain for the mother, but they can and do get to the baby. Their effects can be lifelong. Drugs should be avoided whenever possible, (neural- apoptosis).

Delivery in the ER

This event rocked my world and eventually changed who I was and what I would dedicate my life to doing. Sometimes in life you get the wonderful opportunity to have that "AHA!" Moment!!! This was in fact, one of these moments for me.

I was working in the hospital when a woman entered the ER holding her stomach and simply squatted down and before anyone could even get to her, she pushed out a perfectly healthy, beautiful baby who required absolutely No interventions or medications for that matter. Both baby and mom were doing great and we all got to bask in the beauty of nature and how normal and natural the process of giving birth should be.

This gave me great pause... for upstairs, we were performing miracles and bringing women back from the brink of death to save them from the tortures of labor and delivery. It dawned on me there and then, that nature wasn't putting these women at risk or compromising their lives... we were! The nature process works, but, we as doctors, were there to save a life when something went wrong... unfortunately, many of the procedures we expose a laboring women to takes her off the natural path and yes, puts her and her baby's lives at risk.

Seeing this woman give birth so naturally and normally made me change my whole process and thinking of the birthing woman... we should be helping and never interfering in a natural, normal, labor and delivery. The simple act of making a woman labor on her back is enough to change the eventual outcome... Don't mess with nature!

One... Two... Multiple Times!!!
(this just keeps happening)

I was used to seeing babies being born in a delivery room with complete general anesthesia care. Babies emerged very lethargic appearing to almost be dead. They were suctioned and giving oxygen immediately. Whisked away to the nurseries before their mothers ever got a chance to hold or see them.

I was an Intern working in obstetrics and got an emergency page to go to the ER. Arriving on the scene there was a lady who was in the act of giving birth. She was fully dressed and conscious and was in a fit of extreme anxiety at the thought that a new life was emerging from within her.

Baby was coming RIGHT NOW!!! She squatted down and with a grunt and a sigh... the baby came out, without the need for any interventions at all. The baby was breathing well and crying lustily. To my surprise, *the baby required no interventions… no iv, no drugs, no suction, no sterility, no need for intubation (resuscitating the baby!)… No prep of any kind! I was in awe of the natural process and started to question what the heck we had been doing upstairs? Drug free… Intervention free… this was simply not possible within the confines of the Hospital upstairs. This reality swirled throughout my mind that this baby and mother had no drugs… why couldn't we do this, on purpose, upstairs? Natural birth was not only possible… it was best for both mother and baby.*

I wound up not cutting the cord, but waiting for the placenta… wrapping it with the baby, and then taking them upstairs to do further procedures.

*This is the routine within the hospital in which we poisoned millions of babies.

The thought crossed my mind that this baby and mother had no drugs… why couldn't we do this upstairs.

Why couldn't we be doing this, on purpose, upstairs?

These acts influenced and changed my life... along with the thousands upon thousands of births I would be present for in the future.

Intern New Britain Hospital, CT

During rounds a resident had all the interns observe a laboring woman who was handling labor remarkably. She was calm, cool, and collected and appeared to be in absolutely no pain at all! This confused the resident and he deduced that this laboring woman must have no nerves in this region at all... Narrow minded indeed! Marion Tompson, one of the Founding mothers of La Leche League tells of a similar incident where everyone under the sun was brought in to witness her handling labor like a trooper!

New Britain Emergency

At the time Vic was not on the OB service, but on ER services, and got a call. "DOCTOR BERMAN, EMERGENCY... COME TO THE ADMITTING OFFICE IMMEDIATELY!" he thought to himself, what kind of emergency could they have down there... a paper cut?

It was like a scene from a play, everyone was standing still and there was the admitting secretary and the husband, and a woman fully dressed, standing there with her baby in her panties... her panties were stretched down and now holding her baby.

While being processed by admitting had some contractions and expelled the baby while fully dressed. Vic proceeded to free this new life from the unlikely environment and simply handed the baby over to the mother... "here's your new baby!" It was just amazing.

Another Birth
There were two examining rooms with an area in-between the two rooms. Vic was examining a patient in one room, while another of his patients was brought into the other room. The nurse examines the second patient.

Vic could hear his patient yell, "DOCTOR BERMAN COME QUICK... THE NURSE SAYS, I'M ONLY 2 CENTERMETERS... I MUST BE MORE THAN THAT!" "YOU EXAMINE ME!"

So, Vic finished with his patient and ran over to the next room, put on a pair of gloves and examined her... sure enough she was two centimeters. (realize that dilation to a doctor is like a clock... indicated how long it's going to be).

While he examined her, another contraction began, and he could feel her transition from 2 to 9 during this one contraction. Vic never saw anything like this before... and he still didn't! But he did feel the expansion and how it can and does happen rapidly, in some situations. The patient went on to deliver within the hour. Total labor was less than 2 hours. Note: this is normal, but not as common. It's a quick birth!

Incident that Nearly Ended His Career

Vic was in medical school and his day started out like many others, but this one had a twist that nearly ended his career.

The hours were grueling and the staff shorthanded. One evening he was left to monitor a patient who was in labor and to deliver the baby when it decided to arrive. For the longest time, everything was normal and there was little to do, but chart the patients progress and wait. Note: this was a medicated patient who was not permitted to labor normally. She was not in control of her own body.

Now it was time for the baby to be born, in a fashion that is not unheard of and actually happens in over 4% of all births. The baby was breech. Now to make things worse, there was a prolapse cord. Meaning the baby had engaged into the birth canal along with the cord wedging between the pelvis and the baby's body.

The problem was that this type of delivery had not been taught to Vic, as of yet. Delivering a breech does have its risks and knowledge is the key along with experience in knowing what to do. A baby emerges like a key going through a lock and you may need to guide and manipulate the baby to get the shoulders out and with a twist, the head.

Being abandoned by the Intern, this baby started to emerge, but Vic was never instructed on what to do! Vic shouted at the nurse to get the Intern, "STAT!" Time ticked by. Vic was helpless in this situation. He could feel the baby move and the cord pulsate... until they didn't. Medications, Pitocin, & restricting the patient to her bed played many roles in creating this now emergency situation.

The Shoulders got lodged and after requesting support and time going by... The worst-case scenario occurred. By the time help arrived (Intern), it was too late!

Vic was mortified... a perfectly healthy baby died in his hands and he had no clue as what to do about it.

A healthy baby succumbed to environment and events that could have been avoided, with proper preparation and training. Vic was overwhelmed and proceeded to storm out of the hospital into winters embrace! Throwing his stethoscope into a snowbank!

"I QUIT!" thought Vic to himself. He was physically, mentally, and emotional distraught! At first, he thought of just continuing to walk away (wearing only scrubs)... luckily it was freezing cold and the weather got the better of him! Maybe nature was looking out for him? Temperature and lack of proper clothing saved his medical career and legacy of thousands and thousands of births.

He eventually made it back into the hospital with a renewed determination to never let something like this happen to him or his patients again!

Note: Today, far less doctors are trained or have experienced a vaginal breech birth. If the patient is delivering breech, then it's an automatic Cesarean.

In the forties they actually rotated the baby to make it breech. For a foot makes a better handle. Podalic Version.

Margaret Hague

Margaret Hague Maternity Hospital was in the facility in New Jersey where I got a tremendous amount of education and knowledge on what to do and what not to do to a pregnant woman while she is in labor and giving birth. Don't get me wrong, I got incredible knowledge and experience handling all kinds of deliveries... unfortunately most of them should have been done another way.

We weren't saving lives we are putting lives at risk and eventually bringing them back from the brink of death and having our patients explain to us how thankful they were for us saving them. If only they knew how we had always been putting them in jeopardy.

Margaret Hague Maternity Hospital introduced Vic to Vaginal Births After Cesareans (VBACs) and how you could try for a VBAC if you had only one prior, but not two or more... this meant an automatic cesarean.

Cesareans were mandatory for a patient with more than one previous cesarean. Also mandatory for a breech presentation and other complications. VBAC's were attempt-ted with a very good rate. Less than 5% wound up with a repeat cesarean.

Residency Margaret Hague

Residency, from 1964-1966 Vic completed only 2 years of a 4-year residency program. He and his classmate had both been selected for this residency program at Margaret Hague Maternity Hospital in Jersey City, New Jersey. This was by far one of the largest maternity hospitals with over 10,000 births a year.

With so many births, Vic was given a great education on nearly all kinds of births. One kind of labor drug was Scopolamine. This was part of the combination of drugs administered to a laboring woman. Upon admission into the hospital they would give their patients a cocktail, if you will, of Scopolamine and Demerol. It wasn't until discussing his training practices that Vic realized that what he was exposing his patients to was the procedure referred to as "twilight sleep". A procedure brought back from Freiburg, Germany. This procedure in Germany came with all the luxuries, elaborate rooms, gourmet foods, a view of the mountains… a dream come true for even a princess. Scopolamine does not prevent pain, just prevents the memories of the torture from it and the need for morphine or Demerol to help. Articles appeared in the *New York Times*, *The Ladies' Home Journal*, and *Reader's Digest* praising Twilight Sleep as the most wonderful experience ever to happen to childbirth.

In 1915 in the United States, one of the founders of the National Twilight Sleep Association, Frances Carmody used this procedure, but died during the birth of her third child. Other women also died during this procedure.

Twilight Sleep took a major hit in its popularity, but was still used, just not referred to by this name… This was a procedure taught to Vic while in medical school, just never referred to by that name.

One could say that this is the, "Jekyll and Hyde" cocktail for birthing. It puts a laboring woman into a state of near unconsciousness, but can make her a raging lunatic, thrashing about and requiring the use of restraints to prevent injuries to herself and staff alike. It is also an amnesiac, which makes the patient not remember labor or delivery, or how she behaved during the procedure. Women would wake in recovery rooms with bruises and marks on their wrists and legs wondering where they came from?

One of the biggest setbacks for Twilight Sleep was the cavalier attitude by hospitals in the U.S. In Germany, this process took a long time and required monitoring and constant supervision to adjust the dosages. In the U.S. we want things now... so it was not uncommon to "up-the-dosage" in the attempt to speed up the process.

My Beautiful Daughter, Sara

Having two sons he would now be blessed with a daughter. This would take place during his Internship at New Britain General Hospital in New Britain, CT.

Because Vic was an Intern in the hospital, he was permitted to stay with Shelly and see his daughter emerge into the world. Something that he missed for the births of his sons.

Vic learned, firsthand, the importance of being there for the birth of your child(ren). The sad part was that this was his third child. There are incredible magical moments that happen when you are present and also being an integral part of the process. Bradley dads aren't spectators, they are participants in the process. As Dr. Bradley was fond of saying, "a husband should be man enough to finish what they start!"

Sara is an Attorney and helps others get prepared to be able to pass the Bar. Her School sends her all over the U.S. making sure that other locations are setup to take on this challenge.

Go West Again, Young Man...

In 1966, Vic uprooted his family and moved out West! Needing a change of scenery and a chance to start anew... he answered an ad in one of the medical trade journals and proceeded to join the Kaiser Permanente Group in Lakewood, California. This was specifically a clinic and he also worked the Kaiser ER in Long Beach.

Separation & Divorce

Although Vic & Shelly moved out to California, they had drifted apart. Eventually they decided to divorce.

ELY

Having moved out west, Vic again saw an ad, this time for the Ely Nevada Medical Group and again moved to a slightly less west location, yet more western in atmosphere.

Vic recalls joining their practice on July 1st and just before the 4th of July weekend celebrations. There was a rodeo going on and a cowboy stumbled into the ER with his arm held tightly and wincing his face profusely. He had a fracture of the midshaft of his humerus bone... he was not laughing though!

Being new to the facility and not having any experience with casting a broken bone, during his previous ER experiences, Vic called upon one of his associates. He was quickly informed to set and cast the bone... and not to bother him again, unless there was a true emergency! With the aid of his nurse, Vic was able to complete his first cast out in the trenches.

Well, he had done one during his medical training, but this was the real world and the patient actually had a broken bone and wasn't merely a fellow classmate used for demonstration and practice.

Ely was a unique experience. Vic recalls seeing more gunshot wounds there than his time on the East coast working at a hospital known to be used by the mob.

All of the doctors in Ely were General Practice (GP's) except for one general surgeon. These were the only doctors in the county and the Ely hospital was the only hospital for hundreds of miles.

Several weeks after he came to Ely, the Nurse Anesthetist, who had done all of the anesthesia care for the group announced that she was going to retire. The practice decided to send one of their own to the University of Utah for a special intensive training course in anesthesia for General Practice Doctors. Now either Vic volunteered or was simply low man on the totem pole and was off to Salt Lake City, Utah.

The program was intense, but Vic accomplished it in record time and with high marks. His fellow associates referred to him as, 'Boy Wonder"!

After returning to Ely, Vic did ALL of the anesthesia for the hospital. His practice was half general practice and half anesthesia, for everyone else. What an Experience!

Moving West... Again!

Although I was almost ready to begin my last semester of my residency program in New Jersey, I got an opportunity to move out west to California and work with Kaiser Permanente. Perhaps I just needed a transition and some new perspective, so I jumped at the chance and uprooted my life and moved across the country to begin A new chapter in my life that eventually would become more like my encyclopedia of events that transpired and hopefully helped the thousands of births I had the honor of being present at.

Not many obstetricians have been as fortunate as I have been in experiencing both sides of the birthing world. I started out knee-deep in the medical model and learned much about how to interfere with the natural process.

Many years later I was able to right a wrong and transition into the world of truly natural husband coached childbirth.

I give an incredible amount of respect and acknowledge that I felt that the talk I had with Dr. Robert Bradley helped clarify my life and put me back on track to finish my residency at Glendale Adventist hospital and to complete my training as an OB/GYN. With this distinction I was able to open my own practice and take on the world.

Dr Robert Bradley became a mentor and a friend and role model for how I was going to start this new concept of a "Birth Center."

Back to California and Beyond

Needing to get back to a "Big City", Vic returned to California. He got credit for all his patient experiences. Then he started to complete a Residency in Anesthesiology at UCLA hospital, but after a while he realized that he really wanted to dedicate his life to obstetrics.

Why and When I Quit Anesthesiology (story)

I was working hard. Anesthesia is not easy -you have to be in the operating room every morning at 7am. And you had a schedule and worked all day. Meetings you were required to attend. Educational training and review to keep abreast of the changing field. Worked under the supervision of an instructor professor of anesthesia teaching you different techniques

One particular day, Vic came into the hospital and checked on the cases for the day. He was to give anesthesia for the chief resident in Obstetrics, who was going to perform an ovarian operation. He had never seen or met this guy before and as soon as he saw him, he said to himself, "I hate him!", "this isn't like you to hate this guy..." and soon realized that in a few moments that psychologically he was doing the job of his dreams and that he belonged in obstetrics!

Perhaps Vic needed this wake-up call to put him on track to his life's work and dedication?

...because he was taking my job.

Almost immediately Vic looked for another position. Within weeks or months, he found it.

I saw an ad in a medical journal for a General Practice Physician willing to deliver babies. "THATS IT!!!" Just the job I was hoping to find!

Sherwood Trimble Group

Vic had stumbled across an ad in a medical journal for the Sherwood Trimble Group. They were looking for a General Practice Doctor (GP) who would also deliver babies. Specifically, a (GP) not OBGYN.

I didn't work for them. They supplied me with everything I needed to start a practice. Covering all of my overhead... and in return I gave them a portion of my income, approximately 40%. This was actually a good deal. I went in with nothing but a stethoscope. Starting my practice with office space, staff, laboratory access, billing department, & Insurance and not even debt for supplies, etc.

Natural Childbirth

Nothing fulfilled me as much as being an obstetrician. To help a new baby emerge into this world, especially when they are to be delivered drug free, episiotomy free, with mom feeling elated, dad protecting his wife and supporting his family, having friends and family there too. It is a great feeling to be of help instead of potentially robbing those who should be at this birth from seeing a joyous one, instead of the medical models' ones.

I truly feel that every woman should and could be given the chance and opportunities to have a Natural childbirth. Bradley is the only way that this becomes a reality to almost all of my patients. I can't begin to quantify how many patients we converted from all other forms of preparations for the most amazing and incredibly gratifying affiliation with the best of them all programs and methods. The Bradley Method®!

I wish all my patients were prepared by taking classes in The Bradley Method®. These were truly the very best births I had the pleasure of attending and lending a hand, instead of grandstanding and removing this miracle event for these parents.

I whole-heartedly recommend for you and all pregnant women to research their options and especially take The Bradley Method® course... 12 weekly classes isn't just a good idea... it's an incredibly important one!

Chance Meeting... Salee B

It was a typical day booked with patients and appointments. Vic was even taking on some patients from a doctor who was on vacation or simply did not make it to work that day.

A patient was sent over to him from the doctor who was not available that day. Salee had an appointment with her regular doctor, but was sent to see Vic instead. Arriving at his office and waiting room, that is what she had to do... wait! Two other patients came and went, Salee was still made to wait.

Finally called into the exam room, Salee was more than a bit agitated! A Nurse herself, she had run out of patience. Just imagine being upset by the staff and circumstance, being asked to undress and wait in a glorified napkin to then meet your future husband?

Although Salee was more than a bit put out, things quickly changed from anger to intrigue. It was quickly made clear that both were divorced. Being that this was a patient, Vic had to put the brakes on this chance encounter and simply let the universe take care of what would be... or would someone step up?

Patient with Grandmother

Around a week later Vic had a mother bring in her daughter who wasn't feeling well. Now this wasn't uncommon, but this time the Grandmother came with them too. Now this also wasn't uncommon, but on this occasion, it was the patient he saw only days ago. To this day, I cannot confirm or deny if this little girl truly had a real reason for the appointment, but conveniently Salee was able to see Vic, not as a patient, but a concerned grandmother.

Salee was not your typical grandmother, she was only beginning her 40's. She had her daughter Doreen when she was barely 16. Doreen now had a little girl of her own, Dawn. Her second daughter Kimberly would arrive Later with Salee present and Vic waiting in the wings.

Again, we are not sure who took the initiative, but someone got up the courage to ask the other to lunch the next day. A date made in heaven? They went to the famous taco stand, Tito's Tacos in Culver City, California. From then it was history! Taking them some time and their other marriages to meet, they finally made a formidable team and were able to take on the medical model of birthing, together.

Union... Stronger Than Steel

Vic and Salee got married on May 5, 1972. Sealing their fates and bonding a partnership not only of love, but the love of birth and the need to change the birthing institution. Got married at a synagogue, Temple Emanuel... there was a small reception at a friend's home. Vic had a beard and the Rabbi was clean shaven. Got many questions as to who was the Rabbi. Vic moved in with Salee and her sons.

Salee brought to the marriage her 3 children, Doreen who was married and had her own family, Kenneth who was 10 and Scott who was 7 years old. Vic Adopted both Kenny and Scott only, because Doreen was already married with one child Dawn and eventually had another, Kimberly, with Vic in attendance for the birth.

My First Experience with The Bradley Method® and a Trained Husband-Coach

Surprises come in all shapes and sizes and I had one that surprised not only me, but my staff and the hospital I worked in. There is a huge difference between a planned medical birth and the occasional accidental deliveries that just happened in other places, mistakenly.

A couple of mine came into Washington hospital to give birth and it was routine and nothing special... I was totally mistaken.

The Husband was loving and supportive and was there for all needs and care of the love of his life and the center of his universe. Labor seemed to go very smoothly. Far less screaming and complaining... just a well- oiled machine working hard to bring this new life into the world.

Eventually the big event was on the horizon. My first impression was that this caring dad was to just hang back and leave the rest to us. He stepped up and was a tremendous help and support to not only his wife, but also to all the staff. He freed us up and was an integral cog in the working machinery of giving birth.

Since he was doing so well the nurses supported this "Hero Husband" and they proceeded to gown him and let him do what he apparently does best. He was the most incredible Mental, Physical, Emotional, and loving support that I had ever experienced. It made sense and we all got on board and rode this ride of support and encouragement.

To this day I still don't know what happened to make everything harmoniously fall in place and make it possible for the most incredible experience and life altering event which gave me a course and cause on how to help pregnant families instead of hindering them.

This enlightened me to the importance of The Bradley Method® and how the "Husband-Coach"* was an instrumental component of successful birthing. Bradley Families Rock!

*Although the husband and father of this baby is very important, you may wish or choose another who will take on the role of the Husband.

Husbandry: the care, cultivation, and breeding of crops and animals.

Glendale Adventist Hospital

After meeting with Dr. Bradley, who strongly suggested that he finish his residency. Vic, just by chance, stumbled across an Obstetrical residency program at Glendale Adventist Hospital in Glendale, California. This gave him the opportunity to complete the residency program he started back at Margaret Hague Maternity Hospital on the East Coast.

During his residency he also saw private patients. Vic was asked to join a prominent Obstetrical practice, once he completed his residency. They let Vic use an office and exam rooms at their facility during his residency program.

Two weeks before Vic was to graduate. Vic was leaving the hospital and headed for the parking lot. Two people were having a discussion in the parking lot and Vic walked over to join them. Vic's "future partner" was talking with another doctor. Pleasantries were made to all. He was now boasting about how he had filled the void in his practice by hiring a "Big Shot Resident" who was a woman. This is how Vic was to learn that his well laid plans had gone up in smoke. Vic never spoke to him again.

A Snake in the Grass

I was finishing up my residency at Glendale Adventist Hospital and was a mere two weeks from officially joining the practice of a Dr. S, who was the chief of Obstetrics at Washington Hospital in Culver City. Dr. S. had a growing practice in Beverly Hills and had sought me out as a partner in his practice.

I was leaving the hospital when I had the mis-fortune of walking by Dr. S and hearing him say aloud how he had just hired a graduate for his practice... a very strange way of informing me that I had been replaced, before even starting.

Later I found out that his wife didn't want me to join his practice because she thought that he would be too busy and have a heart attack and die.

Although this was like a knife stuck into my back... in hindsight was probably the motivation and ultimately the best thing that could have happened to me.

*Instead of continuing in the medical model of the day...
I was able to strike out and become the model for all
Birth Centers today!*

*Although I'm not ready to thank Dr. S for being so
rude... I must admit that things worked out in my favor
and for that matter... the thousands of babies I
delivered in-spite of him.*

Now what to do???

Vic was practically thrown to the street and he did not
feel like returning to Sherwood Tremble and their
system. It was a great fit at the beginning of his career,
but losing 50% of his income and being under their
restraints did not fly anymore.

Fortunately, the hospital administrator at Washington
Hospital either took pity on him or was just doing a
great service. Either way Vic was given access to a
converted patient room that would work as his new
office space. The perfect arrangement to be inside of
the hospital and also have space to see his patients.
This worked very well, until a backlash started from
other doctors in the hospital, complaining that this
arrangement was not fair to them.

Gets the Boot... Again

Again, kicked to the streets! Vic was able to find temporary office space with a group on Washington Blvd. This arrangement worked well during the renovation of another location on Washington Blvd that would become the NACHIS location for his office space... later it would be developed into the NACHIS Birth Center.

Asilomar

In December of 1972, Vic & Salee took The Bradley Method® Teacher Training being held at Asilomar in Pacific Grove, California. A beautiful location. Ideal for their training and opportunity to advance the bonds and relationship that was growing with the Hathaways… their entire family.

This was a four-day intensive training process that helped Vic & Salee beyond imagination. Not only did they get time with the Hathaway's, but eventually Dr. Bradley, Dr. Tom Brewer, and Marian Tompson… just to name a few. This was a melting pot, if you will, of contributors to the advancement of childbirth… we all know that it has always been a roller coaster ride and rational and incredible people need to place the train back on its track now and again.

The conference grounds are nestled inside of one of nature's retreats. Wildlife abound from squirrels to racoons, and deer aplenty. Trees throughout the grounds and the Pacific Ocean within sight and just a few minutes' walk to her shores. If you were lucky enough to score a corner room, it even had a fireplace. Some rooms looked out to the Pacific Ocean and others to the forest you were now part of. A tranquil retreat, but the conference rooms were brimming with eager couples and staff alike.

During a break, Vic would head off to the wharf and pick up shrimp that he would bring back to his room and cook in the fireplace. The conference would go past 10 pm, but a treat of shrimp and shish kabobs routinely happened.

Dr. X (a patient's worst nightmare)
Vic was so taken with the groups we drew to us that he just couldn't help himself and would bring a rather unique opportunity to our groups. He would disguise himself and be presented as an honored doctor guest to field questions from our eager trainees. This is how Dr. X (his alter ego, Medical overload) was derived and made a part of those particular workshops. Everyone had a blast and it really was enlightening and gave the group a chance to think outside the box and look at both sides of pregnancy issues.

If it had not been for this Training with The Bradley Method, Vic & Salee both agree that their venture with NACHIS would never have been as successful or rewarding. Too often people choose the quick route or the one with the least resistance. The Bradley Method is by far the greatest form of childbirth education and has made an indelible mark upon the earth and with nearly every pregnant couple today. If your husband, partner, or others attend the birth of your baby... this is indirectly because of The Bradley Method. Perhaps the greatest strides in childbirth today have in many ways been implemented, advanced, or simply humanized because of the great efforts still forged on by The Bradley Method® and all their incredibly talented and dedicated instructors and staff.

The Bradley Method® Teacher Training

This was a chance to be entrenched with likeminded people who you were around morning, noon, and night. The day would begin in a manner of speaking with a Dinner bell or rather the breakfast bell ringing out and notifying all that it was time to gather together for a meal. People would leave their sleeping rooms and make the short trek through the woods and down a road to the dining hall which served meals and had seating areas for the different conference areas. This bell rang out at 7 am.

You would enter the dwelling and get in line to make your way through a corridor that had choices available for your eating desires. Usually three protein choices and other vegetables and carbs to be had. Cafeteria style. To say that most were fans of the food, would be an understatement, but it was hot, brown, and for the most part... plenty of it! This probably inspired the after-conference gatherings where shrimp and shish kabobs from a local shop were procured.

Vic remembers fondly the quality time with Bradley, Bresky, and others.

Bradley was instrumental in getting Vic to complete his residency and became a specialist in OBGYN. Dr. Arnold Bresky was head of Obstetrics at Westpark hospital, in California. This inspired Vic, but eventually, he was going to be working outside of the hospital environment and having an ally, like Bresky, was incredibly reassuring.

Brewer Nutrition

Vic also met a mentor of his, Dr Thomas Brewer. Tom brought light to the necessity of a protein diet... a high protein diet was preferable. Tom was a visionary and realized that you have to take any change as a victory. He would go to clinics on his days off and counsel women how simple changes to their diets could make a Big difference. He would say, "If you're going to have a candy bar, at least get one with nuts!"

Brewer especially counseled high-risk patients over 35, medical deformities, health conditions, Diabetes, epilepsies, thyroid issues, high blood pressure, poor nutrition, etc. Age was not a factor for being high risk. Medical reasons, physical.
Brewer advised them to stop taking drugs, no smoking, take Bradley classes, have good nutrition, and the need to want and desire a drug free birth!

Tom Brewer partnered with The Bradley Method® and together they changed the world and how women were treated, when it comes to nutrition and how he knew how to reverse the trend of small babies, unhealthy pregnancies, and high-risk mothers.

In part, years later this contributed to the success of NACHIS and later on Birth Centers everywhere. Advising a pregnant woman of the necessity of a Balanced Diet consisting of 80-100 grams of Protein a day is a key component of not just preventing, but also reversing some "high-risk" patients to become "low-risk" again… GAME CHANGER!!!

Dr Thomas Brewer's dedication to prenatal nutrition has perhaps done more for the pregnant woman and her growing baby than any other contribution to pregnancy. A healthy, nutritionally sound woman & baby are more able to endure and succeed despite roadblocks they may encounter.

Washington Hospital Film Showing

It was not uncommon for the Hathaway's, who created The Bradley Method, to have film showings in hospitals and other facilities whenever they could. One such film showing was being held at Washington Hospital in Culver City, California.

A patient was in labor and wanted to see the film. She was wheeled into the showing and got a crash course on giving birth without the need for drugs or most interventions. This was so motivating and exciting to her and her husband that they went back upstairs and utilized the techniques shown in the film.

Introduction to
The Bradley Method®

I had been receiving mail asking me to join the Lamaze Method as a professional.... But what really confused me was that I was also getting mail saying that I should join the "real Lamaze Method", regions and groups were fighting with each other.

Walking through the halls of Brotman hospital, out of the corner of my eye a flyer to come to a film showing and meeting with Dr. Bradley was posted on the wall. Intrigued I wanted to hear his perspective on the "Lamaze Method"... for surely, he was there to speak about them.

After about thirty seconds I realized he was not speaking about "Lamaze", but rather a method of childbirth that works and how exuberant he was about sharing this knowledge and concept. How women can walk out of the delivery room, nurse on the delivery table, have their husbands not only with them, but active participants in the whole process. He exclaimed how a husband should be man enough to finish what they start.

This awoke in me the passion and desire to make it possible for every woman to give birth naturally!

Not only did I hear from my future mentor, I also got to see a film that showed the process and how truly successful every birth should and could be.

Afterwards I got to speak with Dr Robert Bradley and we became instant friends and fellow champions of the unborn.

He inspired me to finish my residency and eventually I created the very first Birth Center EVER! This was the seed that led us to the NACHIS Birth Center.

Thank You Marjie & Jay Hathaway and Dr. Bradley... you changed our lives!

NACHIS

You need to understand that when Vic and Salee Berman contemplated letting a woman labor and birth outside of the hospital, that was considered, "undesirable to have a baby outside of a hospital, not safe, and downright Dangerous!!! Let's not confuse hysteria with the reality that women have been giving birth for thousands, if not millions, of years, and if it weren't possible... None of us would be here today!

Office & Location
This, in part, was done because of losing his office space at Washington hospital in Culver City, CA. Vic was well liked and was given access to office space within the working hospital. At first this was a dream situation. To see patients and to be able to perform procedures in the same building. One of the patient rooms was converted into an office for Vic to see patients and do his paperwork.

Unfortunately, this would be short lived. Other doctors complained about how unfair this arrangement was and eventually the administration asked him to find an alternate location for his office space. In so doing, inadvertently gave rise to the first ever "Birth Center" in the world.

The Term, "Birth Center", was coined by Victor Berman and Jay Hathaway. Other environments had been tried and used for birth, but they racked their heads together and for the very first time used this term based the criteria they eventually established.

On Washington Blvd. in Culver City, California an unassuming office location would be transformed to possibly the most successful and incredible childbirth experience, which rivaled and, in many ways, surpassed the home birth experience. They tried to incorporate all the amenities of home with the added safety of having medical devices on hand, baring routine medications. Also, they were merely blocks away from the hospital. All these components made for the ideal facility to labor and give birth. With thousands of births... this must be true!

At first this was to simply be an office for Vic's patients to be seen. But somehow there was always the underlying concept to help the laboring couple have an experience that would change their lives forever. They had an exam room which included a queen size bed... why in the world did they need this? Turns out that it was the perfect labor and birthing bed with enough room for mom, dad, and even the occasional doctor (to sit on and deliver the baby) and siblings to congregate in a very comfortable environment.

Their waiting area just so happens was modified to include a play pen or area that was sunken into the floor with lots of seating and floor space to coral the littles ones with lots of toys, books, at confinement to help entertain and keep everyone happy.
The Birth Center even had a washer and dryer to take on any situation.

This location was possibly chosen to be strategically located between Brotman Hospital and Tito's Tacos just blocks away in opposite directions.

Vic's winks when he explains that the first births at their locations simply happened when a patient came in for a routine checkup and wound up laboring and staying for their birth. Well, the first births were so very successful that they knew that they had the perfect concept in play and would need to name the incredible venture. Salee says that she had a dream about this.

But What Does NACHIS Mean?

One night, Salee had a dream about it and was delighted to wake up with the idea of calling their practice and eventual Birth Center, NACHIS! This was short for the Natural Childbirth Institute. Also, it has a connection to the Yiddish word, Nachas... meaning that you are happy and proud, especially of one's children's accomplishments. An example is what you feel when a woman gives birth naturally to her children.

Hand of Fate

They were seeing patients with only an exam in mind or office treatment. On one particular day, a patient came in for an exam. She was in labor, but did not want to go to the hospital just yet. Everyone decided it was a nice day and simply hang out at the office, which was more home like and when it was time, they would all proceed to the hospital together.

Vic & Salee continued with their appointments at their office and checked in on the laboring woman during the day.

She was progressing nicely, and no one saw the need to transfer to the hospital just yet. Labors can take hours or even days... so no one was in a rush.

This couple was able to labor on queen size bed in the, "minor surgical room", ...why on earth would there be a queen size bed in there? Perhaps there was notion brewing within them that this might become a huge benefit. Vic still says that they did not know that it was going to be used this way.

Since all was going smoothly and this Bradley couple were well trained and laboring well... things just proceeded!

When delivery seemed close, the time came for an attempt to transfer to the hospital. Upon hearing this, the laboring woman simply said, "why can't I just stay here?" Great question indeed!

When it was almost time to transfer to the hospital, the laboring woman simply asked, "Why can't I just stay here and have my baby?"

Eventually the inevitable happened, as it has happened for women for thousands of years! They gave birth in a healthy, happy, environment where everyone was calm, cool, and collected. There was no need for heroics or medicines. Just the loving embrace of mom & dad to greet this new life and welcome them into this world.

NACHIS was even instrumental for the birth of Marjie and Jays 6th child, Ann. Marjie labored at home and was planning on a home birth, but when things did not progress, as hoped. They decided to make their way to the Birth Center which was minutes away from the hospital. They did labor at the NACHIS Birth Center and eventually give birth to their daughter Ann, with a host of on lookers... nearly 18 in total!

It turned out to be a compound presentation with Ann's arm making it difficult to be birthed. Once the elbow, arm and head emerged, it was smooth sailing from there. She was nearly 10 lbs. at birth and gestated for over 10 months. It's not right to rush things! Nature and her mom's body took care of her. The placenta was healthy and normal and could have gone longer, if needed. But the placenta has its own life cycle... it is the only complete organ in the human body that does so. Growing and dying separate from any other organ of a human body.

Of course, after this long day... we all got Tito's and headed back home! Ann's very first feedings were enhanced with the flavors of Tito's Tacos!

Countless celebrities walked their hallowed halls

Ted Lange, Mariette Hartley, PJ Soles, Dennis Quaid, just to name a few...

If you had a wonderful birth at the NACHIS Birth Center, please submit your birth story at info@BradleyBirth.com. We would love to share these with the world and maybe at the next printing you might be included in the revised edition.

NACHIS... *Sounds more like an appetizer then what it was!*

Birth Center

I have the unique honor of being one of two people who coined the phrase "Birth Center". This was the brainchild of myself and Jay Hathaway. Together we came up with this new concept and with the aid of my wife Salee were able to open the very first Birth Center in the entire world. There were perhaps other facilities that were outside of the hospital, but no one had ever used the term "Birth Center" before.

Much of my education on the natural process came from spending incredibly valuable time with Marjie and Jay Hathaway along with Dr. Bradley, Dr. Brewer, & Marian Tompson of La Leche League... Just to mention a few of my heroes.

So I want to take a moment and thank Marjie and Jay Hathaway in particular for meeting with me and Salee on so many occasions and bringing us into their home and family and giving us not only their ears but shoulders to lean upon to help us to mastermind a process on how to give birth naturally... Without drugs in an environment that was as close to being at home as could be and still a medical type environment.

Did I mention that The Bradley Method® and Marjie and Jay Hathaway took us under their wings and gave us a foundation of incredible knowledge and friendship and the expertise along with a professional avenue of being able to record and document our progress and facility through some of the very first films about birth? In part this helped put us on the map and opened the doors for an amazing amount of celebrity clientele seeking us out to have the very best births possible.

Japanese couple (NACHIS)

In the days before ultrasound, unexpected twins were not uncommon. Sometimes even with ultrasound.

First baby delivered... but her belly did not deflate, and it dawned on them that it was twins! Salee exclaimed "Vic, watch out for twins!" Putting his hand on her abdomen realized that there was another.

The laboring woman's Husband was an interpreter, spoke 5 languages. He was so excited and spoke in his native language... until it dawned on him that Vic doesn't speak Japanese and proceeded to change to English. "You say twins... second better be a boy as the first was a girl..." now there would be two girls. They already had a girl at home and the father was hoping for a boy to round out the group. Both keepers!!! and they did not throw one back!

She appeared to be the same size as her prior pregnancy and it's still a mystery on where she kept the second baby.

They were identical twin girls! In spite of wanting a boy, the dad was very happy with his twin girls.

Vic delivered 20-30 twins over the course of his career. Twins club!

Pray for a Partner

Dr Bradley used to say, "Pray for a Partner!" It was so hard to find someone with like mind and attitude to rely on. For years Vic would send letters to OB residency programs both in US and Canada. The responses were few and horrifying. "I'll do any kind of childbirth you want." "Natural, of course, but will give drugs whenever requested. They had complete misunderstanding of what Natural Childbirth was and were just giving a "BS" response to get the job. Now he understood what Bradley was referring too.

The medical model and training are so intense and focused on saving a life instead of only being there to assist a pregnant patient that they simply have forgotten that the act of giving birth is a truly natural, normal event that the majority of women can and should be allowed and encouraged to do. It is BEST for mother and baby!*

Dr Delee is credited as being the father of modern obstetrics. He had a notion that all women needed to have a routine collection of procedures to be performed on them before the birth of their babies. These included but not limited to... receive an episiotomy, use forceps, and of course to be medicated. He even had the notion that women were like a salmon and were simply used up during the process of giving birth. ...where do they come up with these things? This is of course ludicrous, and we will say it here and now that that is absolutely not the case!

Perhaps more damage was done in the name of science and procedures instead of letting nature run her course? The United States is by far more invasive and aggressive than most countries. And still has one of the worst outcomes? Is this because of the overuse of procedures, medications, technologies, etc? <u>DAMN RIGHT IT IS!!!</u> Don't get us wrong, it is wonderful to be living in a time where there are drugs, tools, procedures that can and do save lives! The unfortunate reality is that they are over-used today! With a nearly 40% Cesarean Section Rate and nearly all births being drugged and having ultrasound... hasn't this gone too far? Shouldn't the USA be number one? Then why are we like 46??? This is shameful and needs to change for the sake of our children... the future!

NACHIS TWO

There actually was a second location for the NACHIS practice. It lasted for only a very short time and there were no births as a result. So, where did they decide to expand their practice?

Vic & Salee loved sailing and getting out on the water. A favorite destination, because of location and beauty was the island of Catalina which was only a short sailing venture away (multiple hours).

Options
Ferry service which takes an hour or a helicopter ride for 15 minutes, were also options. 41 miles from Marina Del Rey to Catalina Island or 29.3 miles from Long Beach or 25.1 miles from San Pedro.

The Ferry service, a high-speed catamaran, which travels at 35 knots and gets you there in about an hour. Or taking their own vessel which was a motorsailer. This takes much longer to accomplish the distance to Catalina. Around 5-8 hours depending on many factors.

The Practice

On one of their visits to the Island they came across the local doctor who delivered babies on the island, but usually transported them to the mainland. He was retiring and posed the notion of Vic & Salee taking over the maternity aspect of his practice. At first, they were very excited and made arrangements for office space.

They did see a few patients, but this was just an impractical venture and after only a few months, took down their shingle on the momentary addition of the NACHIS Catalina Experience.

Love for the Water

Not only does Vic have a love to be on the water, but also to be in it! As a little boy he would put fear into passersby as he played on the row boats on their pond and then proceed to jump and frolic in the water. This appeared to be upsetting to neighbors as they rushed over to complain to Vic's mother about this water boy and how they were concerned. Vic's mother never worried about Vic's abilities and his love for the water.

All through his life, he had this connection and need to be near, on, or in the water. This love was definitely part of his swimming activities and eventually leading him to learn and be a certified Scuba diver. His boat was even equipped with an air compressor to refill the tanks of air for diving adventures.

18-20 would go skin diving and use a spear gun to explore the deeps of the waters. In Echo Lake, Brandon, VT crystal clear water. Shot bass primarily.

163

Vic was able to extend this love to his children, especially David who would go diving with him off the coast of Catalina.

You may wonder how in the world did Vic have the time for all his adventures... turns out that with his patient load, there would be windows of opportunities to expand his knowledge and passion for many different aspects that make him who his is.

Vessels
Rowboats and canoeing in his youth.
Rowboat with small concrete brick, upside down oar, and sheet for a sail. Makeshift sailing vessel. Taught him how to catch the wind.

Little boats "Sea Snark" smaller than a canoe (11 ft). Styrofoam 30 lbs. during residency in NJ (30) used in bay near where they lived, NJ bay. Sailing fun for one person. Two if you want to get wet,

Newport 16 had a cabin, trailer. California

Erickson 27 Marina Del Rey, Catalina,

Nauticat 31 "Salee B" single hull diesel motorsailer

Catamaran "Double Chai" dual diesel motorsailer

Somehow or another, Vic was asked to work the Florida sailboat show. He had met a blind man whose father builds catamarans. Vic worked the show for a week as a salesman. In part, payment was discounted for service rendered for the purchase of their vessel, the "Double Chai". Flew to Great Britain to see it before it was shipped. Sailed a similar vessel on the English Channel. Shipped as cargo and going down to Long Beach.

Catamaran 32, Double diesel "Double Chai", used engine 3-4 hours a day to keep batteries charged, freshwater system reverse osmosis system. Could be a real home. Sold in Florida.

Catalina 27. Lived on with Mookie a couple months.

California to Florida 5k mile journey. Filled up 5 times during the excursion.

When very young, vacationed in Mexico with his family and they rented a sailboat. First time sailing with a big boy boat!

Just Me and the Open Waters...

Vic was around 5 years old when a concerned neighbor rushed in to tell his mother that Vic was jumping out of a small boat into the lake next to the lodge. This lady was very concerned, "how could anyone let a small child do this without any supervision?" Well, Vic went to the water as a fish to the sea... they were one and lived in harmony. Vic was a strong, capable swimmer and had been so for a very long time.

In retrospect, this would not be considered good parenting today, but back then parents would scoot their children out the door and would not expect to see them for hours or until the sun was going down and food was on the table.

His time on the lake, rivers, etc. just increased his love for the water and one day would be a sea captain and sail all the way from Los Angeles to Florida. Traversing the Panama Canal and navigating from the Pacific Ocean to the Atlantic. A dream that would take him a decade to achieve & complete and with incredible losses along the way.

Vic is a U.S. Coast-Guard licensed Captain and certified Scuba diver. The lodges he grew up at afforded him great exposure and time in and on the waters. He would jump from the rental boats into the water, or sail around on the ponds or lakes.

In New Jersey he had a Snark sailboat which he could drive to the shore, off the Statue of Liberty and enjoy the Hudson River with a view of lower Manhattan on one side and to the side, Lady Liberty herself. Vic eventually transitioned into an Ericson 27 sailboat, "Salee B", and then the "Double Chai"

Oxymoron... Jumbo Shrimp

Vic & Salee and their son Scott were out taking the Salee B on a test run before there epic journey. They were sailing off the coast of Mexico and came upon a fishing trawler with large nets hanging off the sides.

Vic approached the vessel and yelled out to the crew and asked if they had any shrimp for sail? Captain responded, "Yes!" and would be willing to part with some for... "WHISKEY!!!" Problem was that they were not drinkers and did not have alcohol on their boat. Vic explained this and the captain then asked for $5 U.S. Vic was more than happy to oblige.

The crew went below and brought back topside a large box filled with refrigerated shrimp. Vic was expecting a small amount for such a little amount of money. What they got was a box full of the most beautiful shrimp imaginable. Not little shrimp but large and extra-large ones. They ate this shrimp morning, noon, and night. Brings to mind a scene from *Forrest Gump* explaining all the ways you can enjoy shrimp! Well, this was their opportunity to try all kinds of ways too.

S...O... S...

Vic & Salee and their son Scott, were out sailing the ocean blue when they had mechanical issues with their boat. Being out in the middle of nowhere they were in serious trouble!

They could not reach land and they were not prepared to be set adrift for too long in these waters and condition.

Eventually they had no choice but to get on the radio and declare an emergency by sending out an S... O... S... meaning Save Our Souls!
There literally were no other vessels near them that could help them in this predicament. What were they to do???

Waiting for a bit, they started to notice that the sea was coming to life... massive movements and waves coming from nowhere... was it the breeching of a whale or King Triton himself emerging from the depths?

Their saviors arose from the sea in a black tubular shaped angel, with small wings extending from a rise along the top of this tube... it was a U.S. Navy submarine springing into action! The Navy boarded their vessel and performed some maintenance on their ship, so they could at least make it back to a port for further adjustments.

Before departing from each other, they were simply asked to never divulge the exact location of their exchange... a small price for saving their lives. GO NAVY!

Salt of the Sea

Vic & Salee loved their time on the water and would try and get out on the ocean whenever they could.

It was getting time for dinner and they decided to prepare a spaghetti dinner.

As any good cook knows, it is important to season the water in which you are going to boil the pasta.

Vic knew this and instead of simply adding a pinch or two of salt to the pot... hoisted water directly from the sea to boil... after all it was already "salty water"!

The pasta cooked as they prepared to enjoy a warm meal out on the ocean.

As they both started to eat the spaghetti... they both had a look and a similar response to whatever this was in their mouths.

It was inedible! It wasn't a little salty... it was over the top salty! They simply could not eat it!

The moral the story is to also have Grubhub, Uber Eats, DoorDash, or Postmates (just anything like these) on speed dial when you try something new!

NACHIS Retirement

"The trouble with retirement is that you never get a day off." – Abe Lemons

Well, as the expression goes... all good things must come to an end. After spending the better part of two decades, Vic & Salee decided it was time to relinquish the torch and start a new chapter of their lives.

As you might know, Vic is a certified Captain of even large vessels and Vic & Salee had a ship that was Yar (a boat that handles with little effort). A good sailing design, quick and capable.) Their motorsailer, The Salee B.

They had a dream of sailing down the coast of California, past Mexico, onwards by Guatemala, El Salvador, Nicaragua, Costa Rico, and making it to Panama to cross through the Panama Canal from the

Pacific Ocean over to the Atlantic Ocean... finally making their way to their new home state of Florida.

Selling their practice to a Midwifery group that promised to keep things going, they felt at ease with their decisions. There was a big party and send off for these icons of the childbirthing community. They were already missed, even though they were still docked.

With their vessel, the "Salee B"... all loaded up with mementos, photos, and nearly all their possessions they set sail. It was incredibly freeing. To have the wind at your back and open ocean in front of you. They basked in the sun and enjoyed their freedom.
Knowing that they would have a lot of down time, they brought with them all their pictures from their practice and were going to work on them during this epic journey.

Zihuatanejo

Making their way down Mexico, they reached the bay of Zihuatanejo. They anchored in the harbor and boarding their dingy, made the short trek to finally step on land again. Heading into town to pick up some supplies and fresh vegetables and fruit. They had not planned on staying in town very long, so they were wearing not much more than swimming attire.

Having had a successful venture into town, they headed back to the bay to unload their bounty of goods.

Reaching the bay, they were confused to not be able to locate their vessel. There was a ship ablaze, but they could not figure out where their ship was... Vic remembered the boat they anchored next to... they could not believe their eyes, it was their boat, the Salee B. that was unrecognizable and barely afloat.

Salvaged a few items that managed to wash up on shore.

Originally, they had no idea how this all began. Later, people came up to Vic & Salee and told the same story of how a group of young boys used a dinghy to get to their boat and later quickly jumped back onto their dinghy and sped away... as flames began to emerge from the boat.

Some local kids had boarded the Salee B. and robbed them blind. Leaving no tracks, they took a flare gun and shot it into the cabin, which set the boat ablaze.

The only thing they could do was watch as their boat finally made its way to the bottom of the bay and to rest next to Davey Jones locker.

The Local Police & Port Authorities came and weren't any assistance. At some point the authorities dragged the skeletal remains of the boat partially onto shore. Vic & Salee weren't allowed access to their once lovely boat.

They went into the office of the Port Authority, with items from their boat setting on his desk. Vic could tell what was coming. The Port Master exclaimed to Vic that their boat had made a mess of his harbor and beach front, and how they were responsible for the cleanup. Vic could tell that he was not going to be walking out with any of the items on the desk. Further, they used their dinghy to help pay for the cleanup.

Vic knew that he wasn't going to be able to leave the office with any of their possessions... with a tear coming to his eyes.

Some onlookers approached Vic & Salee and offered them shelter at their home, while they were dealing with this mess. The kindness of strangers still moves Vic today.

They only had a few pesos (money) to their names and not much of anything else. They made their way back into town and did the only thing they could think of... they called Marjie & Jay Hathaway! Veteran travelers they knew they, one. Could cry on their shoulders, and two that Jay would know how to help them... they were right and the Hathaway's sprang into action and made arrangements to get them some money and a way to get home.

Although they had a way to get out of Mexico, it still had its challenges. They boarded a bus and made their way to the airport. This was not a bus ride, like you would have in the States... instead they were sharing the ride with the locals, along with their livestock... To say that there was a unique odor would be an understatement! But they made it to the airport and finally got back to family and friends.

NACHIS Stories

During their voyage on the "Salee B", Vic & Salee took with them the cards, letters, pictures, etc. from all their patients while operating the NACHIS Birth Center... They Burned up or wound up at the bottom of the ocean.

If you were one of the lucky ones to utilize this great institution and have your story, pictures, etc. Please send them in and we will put them all together for another edition of this book series.

We look forward to hearing and seeing your stories and thank you for sharing in advance.

Send to AAHCC Box 5224, Sherman Oaks, CA 91413 or Email to Info@BradleyBirth.com

Second Chance

After losing almost everything...

Vic & Salee had returned to the States after having a very trying experience.

They had packed on board all the pictures, letters, memories of their time cultivating the NACHIS Birth Center. Salee knew there would be a lot of down time and this would be a great activity while they sailed their way to Florida.

Everything was lost! Burned up or sank to the bottom of the Sea.

Although they had retired from their practice in California, they were basically relocating to Florida and would start up a new site once they had gotten re-established. A condition of selling their Practice was to not open another Birth Center near their old one. Florida is all the way across the country.

So, what were they to do? Vic had a lot of training and experience as an ER doctor.

Vic landed a job as an ER doctor in Banning, California. A chance to get back on their feet and decide what they were going to do... in the long run.

They made Banning their home for a year, but eventually made their way back to their roots. Brotman Hospital is home to Vic and they decided to open up an office at the Brotman location. They had medical buildings next to the hospital, which made it an ideal location to start anew.

Now Vic & Salee never opened another Birth Center. But they did have an office suite with plenty of room to see patients, have classes and lectures, & just in case supplies on hand to deliver a baby, if the opportunity presented itself.

Alice Garrido
Alice Garrido, a valued friend and assistant to them throughout the years and locations.

Alice was a Nanny for a patient of theirs. The patient made it known to them that Alice had legally immigrated to the states and had been a Nurse in Argentina. Alice's husband had a television repair shop. Like many others had come to the States in hoping to make a better life and was only working as a nanny to make ends meet until she could be licensed in the U.S. Salee especially, reached out and gave her a job and helped her study for the exam.

Alice passed the exam and stayed on with Vic & Salee through the location changes. Alice & Salee made an incredible team. Salee was a Certified Nurse Midwife and Alice was her ever faithful companion who shadowed Salee and made their home-birth option a success.

Barbara Kalmen

Blessed with many wonderful nurses who worked with them through the years, Barbara Kalmen was one of them. Not only did she help at NACHIS she was also employed at Brotman Hospital and was able to assist with Vic's patients at both locations.

While having a great career in nursing, Barbara longed for more and sought out an opportunity most wouldn't have thought of.

She was reaching a junction that would forever change the course of her life. The military has a cut off for people wishing to enlist... with both feet she dove in and had an incredible career in the Air Force. Achieving the rank of Lt Colonel, Retired.

While on active duty and stationed at Edwards Air Force base in the Mojave Desert, which is 100 NE of Culver City. She was pregnant and made arrangements to get time off and had her third child at NACHIS.

During active labor, they traveled to NACHIS, which more than likely took over two hours to get there.

She had a wonderful birth and was thrilled to be home again at NACHIS.

Our Staff

We had many wonderful people working for and with us through the years. They all were tremendous assistants and we appreciated their dedication to our visions and for helping us make it possible for our patients to achieve the births of their dreams.

Backup

To be a successful Midwife you need to have backup. Salee not only had backup from an Obstetrician... she was also sleeping with him. Being married to Vic had many advantages.

Vic learned through the countless births they both attended that to be a good doctor, you needed to keep yourself occupied or at least... "keep thy hands in your pockets!" a saying Dr Bradley was fond of. But also tinkering with a new camera was never a bad idea. At many births we would catch Vic learning the ends and outs of his new toy and hobby.

OFFICE

The New office location was in a building, Brotman Physicians Plaza. With offices for Vic & Salee, a large waiting/gathering area, Reception area, Exam rooms,

Bathrooms, etc. It was a very nice location with most of the amenities of NACHIS Birth Center.

They knew that they would not open another Birth Center, but they did have the notion that the occasional patient just might labor and eventually give birth there.

Birth Stories, Lonquich Family

The Lonquich's are incredible people who are extremely supportive and even advisors to The Bradley Method. Paul is an MD and Professor and Vickie is a Physician's Assistant.

When they got pregnant, of course they took The Bradley Method 12 weekly classes, to prepare for the arrival of their first child.

Being that they are part of our extended family and well... we were driving them to the Berman's Office, made it convenient to be able to be present at the birth.

They were living in Sylmar, California, at the time and we got a phone call asking if we wouldn't mind taking them to Vic & Salee's office. We were thrilled to help out, besides we had a 15-passenger van with a seat or

187

two removed for the trek, which made it an ideal transportational vehicle.

Loaded up, we carefully got onto the 405 freeway (the busiest freeway in the world... at least was) and made the trek to Culver City that night.

Grandparents- Gene and Peggy, Herb & Louise "Lou", along with Marjie, James, & Ann Hathaway, Vic & Salee, Alice Garrido, Bill Fong, and Paul & Vickie had all made the journey to the office to be present for the birth.

Ann and Paul had had talks about how one prepares for the arrival of a new baby... they agreed to have a cooler on hand with Dove bars at the ready! Dark chocolate, of course.

As things progressed, Peggy peeked her head in just to check, Marjie without missing a beat asked Peggy to get a washcloth... from then on, she was part of the team and was taking a role in the birth.

This baby really wanted to be born. We can say this because of what we discovered at the birth!

The birth went without incident, up until Vic examined the placenta and was shocked to discover what we were all looking at. Now this baby really wanted to be born, for imbedded into the placenta itself, was a Copper 7. An IUD that had been assumed to have fallen out years before.

Paul did catch and not deliver his son. We feel the term catch is a more accurate way of expressing what should happen. A mother and baby do most of the work.

Mom and baby were doing great and the sun had risen. All were in the mood for breakfast, perhaps no one as eager as Vickie. She had just given birth and they waited for the placenta and to be signed off that all was well... we all headed out to Ships Coffee Shop and had Breakfast.

Now we were a fair-sized group with a little baby to boot. The waitress came over and asked how old the baby was... without hesitation, Vickie exclaimed, "a couple hours old!" The waitress was perhaps a bit shocked, but quickly fell in love with him and took all our orders.

Second Time Around

Now Vickie is one of those women who should have a hundred babies.

Again, we were honored to be asked to take them to the office. So, we headed over to do a repeat of their first birth. All was the same except this time with brother Brian with us in a car seat instead of Vickie's tummy.

Reaching the office. We barely got Vickie out of the elevator and onto a bed before she preceded to birth her second child Blake. Simply 3 or 4 contractions and it was all over.

Three Times a Charm

For their third baby, Vic & Salee were out of town and being very comfortable with the process and the fact that Paul is an MD who has delivered countless births himself, they felt confident enough to have their third baby at home.

Paul has a strong medical background and needs to intervene; it's how he was trained as a doctor. So, when they were preparing for the imminent birth, Paul told Marjie Hathaway how he had his trusty bulb syringe at the ready and was going to jump in and us it as soon as he could.

Well the birth happened, and everyone was delighted and basking in the afterglow of seeing a new life emerge into this world. It was not rushed, and Paul was too entrenched with this new life and took his time and just watched and observed the natural birthing process.

Now about 45 minutes had elapsed since the birth. Marjie couldn't just let it alone and spoke up to Paul reminding him that he didn't get to use his cherished medical device. Paul sprang into action and looked at the syringe and was about to reach for it when Marjie calmly said, "don't you dare!" The baby was doing beautifully and there was absolutely no reason to use this device. The Fetal Heimlich Maneuver did its job and vacated the mouth, nose, throat and lungs of mucous and liquids upon the expulsion of the baby. Don't mess with Mother Nature!

The Lonquich family now added a baby girl to their clan. She was a beautiful red-headed little girl and would soon have them all wrapped around her little fingers.

UPDATE

Following in the family tradition. Their first-born son, Brian is now a double board-certified Doctor of Pediatrics and Internal Medicine. Married to Erica and living in Houston, Texas.

Second born son, Blake is a technician for Amtrak and makes one heck of a commute every day.

Third born, daughter Brianna is also follow-ing in the family medical endeavors and is a lab technician working on becoming a PA, like her mom.

The Joy of Natural Birth

Look forward to the birth experience, don't be afraid of it! This may be the most important & significant experience of your life! No matter how much you think you know, you will still learn & experience new things, surrounding every birth!

Here I was, I a graduate of medical school, MD, internship first year including OB, two years residency, advanced training in OB, three years private practice... mostly OB, had delivered my first 200-300 babies!!! What could I learn from a training program from The Bradley Method? How to relax, exercise, positions, dealing with contractions! What to expect? The importance of the experience!

You cannot appreciate the natural process, if anesthetized! You will miss so many Magical Moments! Look forward to it! Again, don't be afraid! Countless pioneering women have gone through The Bradley Method and have confirmed and solidified all the techniques and training a mother needs today to have a Happy Birth-Day! Bonding with your baby, Love, taking care of yourself, importance of high protein balanced diet, necessary weight gain, exercise, husband (or other companion) who are trained and prepared for this unique birth, above all to prepare for your expanding family! Birth is not a spectator sport and the mothers get no substitutions!

Personal Note: I learned! Bradley changed my life! Changed my medical practice!

I was trained to be a "life-saver". That all women were incapable of delivering without heroic efforts, equipment, drugs, and technology. Experiencing my first couple prepared with The Bradley Method was an incredible life-altering experience. I will be forever grateful for partnering up with this amazing program! This showed me that, medically speaking, we had it all wrong! We were there for the rare times that interventions were required! That a prepared couple should not only be given the chance, but all the support necessary to avoid interventions whenever possible. As Dr Bradley said, "a trained husband can do more for a laboring woman than any amount of medication!" This was radical to me, but Bradley had it right!

I cannot emphasize enough the importance of The Bradley Method® and Natural Childbirth. Bradley babies start life with the best advantages available, during a normal healthy pregnancy, labor, and delivery.

Victor Berman, MD

Walking on Water

Vic & Salee had a lovely home in Culver City. In the backyard was a pool and a fishpond that even had a small bridge running over the top of it. Fish galore made this their home and Vic sometimes fed them dry dog food... hence the reason we referred to them as dog fish. There was a shade tree that protected the pond and overhung the pool just a bit.

One day, the dogs started barking at a squirrel, which made him run up the tree. This squirrel had been tormenting the dogs and now found himself in a very precarious situation. This squirrel kept moving further and further out on a branch, mocking the dogs in the process. Eventual he proceeded out too far and fell into the pond!

Now I'm not sure as to the swimming skills of this little guy, but I just might believe that he could fly and in part walk on water. For as soon as his body hit the water, he flung into action and bolted from the scene. Out of harm's way, he turned his little head in discontent and went off to find another adventure.

Our Son Kenny & Family

Salee's First son, Kenneth, graduated from Vermont College in Hotel Management. He moved to Mammoth, California and became a Popular Ski instructor. Karen & Kenny met on the slopes and married. They have a son Michael, who was on track to be an Olympic athlete. It was because of a bout with Mononucleosis (Mono) that derailed Michael's Olympic dreams.

Pregnant with their only child, they opted to make the journey to the NACHIS Birth Center to be delivered by the Grandmother, Salee. Vic simply took pictures... and of course, backup!

Michael was born, but within a day or two had indications of a medical condition which was alarming. This seemingly healthy child had an incredible case of jaundice! This was perplexing to all... baby was healthy, but was yellow. After consulting and working with some of the greatest minds in pediatrics, they came to a conclusion... Living at an altitude of 9000 feet and coming down to sea level to have the baby, caused the Jaundice condition. Jaundice is caused by the breakdown of red blood cells.

Normally a baby is born with a surplus of red blood cells and is broken down after the first few days. And when they break down, a cast of yellow color is visible in the skin. Jaundice by itself is not a disease, but a description of the coloring of the skin. Because of the altitude both mother and baby had extra cells. Sunlight is nature's way of taking care of this condition of excess. Both mother and baby did just fine! Salee was the one to figure it out though!!!

Change of Course

Their hotel was near the airport. Vic's mother was living at a retirement community. At the hotel the parking lot was nearly full. They didn't want to walk through the parking lot, so they drove around until a space opened up near a brightly lit side door entrance... there was nothing at the front of the facility.

Salee gets out of the car and heads for the door. A car had been following them, but they assumed that they too were looking for a parking space.

Salee could hear footsteps and then a guy runs up to Salee, grabbing her purse. Her reflexes went into action and without hesitation, with both hands yanked her purse back from him. Vic ran to Salee's aid, but slipped and fell, injuring his knee and back. Vic's knee was bloody. Guard comes up and says, "I'm gonna get them!". Police report was filed... but they did not go to the hospital.

They came back home to California, but Vic's back was still hurting. He saw an Orthopedist and Neurosurgeon... diagnosis, slipped disk and recommended surgery.

Several weeks later they visited his mother again and Vic's back was really hurting. They decided to have surgery on his back.

Successful surgery, but he was never right again. Could not stand and perform a surgery himself. Just seemed to be a good time to retire on disability. The final straw that possibly broke the camel's back... kind of forced retirement.

Double Chai

The word "Chai' translated from Hebrew to English means "Life."

Vic's daughter Sara was pregnant with twins. Salee and Vic had retired and were living in Florida. They made the trek out west to be close at hand. Sara would have her babies at a hospital in Beverly Hills, California.

Everything started out as the picture-perfect birth and environment. Sara labored with her husband and eventually gave birth to Daniel, a healthy baby boy. Everyone was delighted.

So, Daniel came out and everyone was basking in this beautiful new life. But then an event would occur to change everything!

Because Sara was having twins, she was considered high risk, so upon admission, the hospital routine insisted on having an epidural connection in place, for the protection of both mother and baby. They do this by inserting the epidural needle and tube into the patients back, into the epidural space and hopefully not puncturing into the spinal canal. This gives the anesthetist a pathway to administer medications at a moment's notice.

So, they placed the epidural, which is only a connection and or pathway to then be able to give drugs and other substances. While doing this they do administer a small dose of medication to confirm that they did indeed place the epidural in the right location and that the patient was responding to this procedure.

Note: an epidural is not a drug, but rather a way of getting drugs to a particular space or area outside of the spinal canal. It is not a spinal. It is a tube which is placed just outside of the dura or epi and if done correctly does not penetrate into the spinal canal. Now the difference between getting an epidural and spinal is crossing through the Dura layers which are actually thin, and sometimes epidurals do become a spinal, by mistake.

Epidurals can include drugs, steroids, etc. Today many procedures include a mixture or "cocktail" of drugs or other substances to these areas.

Sara had labored and gave birth to a natural born first baby, Daniel. Right after delivery, the anesthesiologist activated the epidural, because this was routine for twins in this hospital, that she did not need or require... or especially want!

This immediately stopped her labor. After an hour, they started Pitocin to right this wrong and proceeded to have contractions with decelerations, which were an indication of distress for the baby. Salee called Marjie Hathaway of The Bradley MethoD® and vented about the situation.

On the surface this may seem to be an act of kindness to let Sara get some relief or respite, but this was not the case and did irreparable harm and damage to this birthing event.

You see, the drugs caused Sara to stop having contractions and instead of simply continuing to have contractions to expel the second baby, it shut down the labor and made it impossible for her to give birth at that time.

The staff would frequently leave them alone, and Vic & Salee were there by her side.

Contractions continued and four hours later, as decelerations became worse, they decided to perform an emergency cesarean, because the baby's heart rate was dangerously low.

Uncle Dr. David Berman to the Rescue

After Julia was born, they whisked her into an isolette to intubate her. The "high risk resident pediatrician" came in and was having a hard time intubating him. His Uncle David stepped in and possibly saved his life! David is a highly skilled and renowned Pediatrician on staff at this hospital.

Sara remained on the delivery table during this whole ordeal, due to the fact that she had an umbilical cord protruding out of her body. Daniel had been born and his cord cut, but the placenta was still attached to the wall of the uterus and would not be expelled until Julia was born or removed from their mom.

So instead of having a truly natural Twin childbirths, she and her baby were now exposed to harmful drugs and would have to wait for them to wear off before her labor could continue.

Her baby now will be exposed to not just a moment of drug exposure, but for potentially hours to come. This stop in labor did continue for hours. Eventually the baby's heart rate declined, and an emergency Cesarean Section was required. Something that probably could have been avoided all together.

Julia was extracted and eventually joined her brother, Daniel. This would occur 5 days later after she was released from the NICU.

Sara joined a truly unique group of women who both have had a natural and medicated delivery for the same pregnancy.

Roger's birth

Vic & Salee had been retired for two years and were living in Florida. They made the journey from Florida to California to be nearby for the birth of their grandson, Roger. They had a conversion van with a couch/bed that was comfortable, and they simply parked it in Ira's backyard to be close at hand.

They had planned to have their baby at Kaiser Hospital.

They all went to bed and tried to get some sleep. Early the next morning they woke up being informed that it was time and that Evelyne was ready to go to the hospital. Vic told Ira that he would pull the van to the front of the house... because it has a bed and would make transport easier.

After waiting for a while, Ira came out and said that Evelyne wasn't able to get up and get to the van. Vic went to go check her and without any equipment or even gloves found that the head was bulging, and they weren't going to make it to the hospital!

Roger was born without incident and they all just basked in the moment. Ira and Evelyne were highly trained in The Bradley Method and they were confident in what was happening and how to give birth. Besides, an Obstetrician and Certified Nurse Midwife were on hand... Vic & Salee.

Vic's son and the baby's Uncle David arrived minutes later, for he was on call to babysit the older brother, Benjamin, who was 2-3 years old at the time. Now David has a thriving practice as a pediatrician. So along with Vic & Salee, they had a medical plethora of knowledge and support.

David arrived about ten minutes after the birth. Completely flustered... had never been to a home birth and exclaimed, we have to take the baby to the hospital and have him checked out. Vic proceeded to say, "I checked the baby... and you've checked the baby... who's better qualified than us?"

You see, after a birth the nurse usually administers shots, blood collections, etc. while a home birth is far less invasive and flows at a more natural rate. Mom and baby didn't just do well... they soared!

In the morning, they went to the hospital to have the baby checked and register the birth. The most difficult thing about a home birth is getting the birth certificate! Arriving at the hospital, they were informed that they couldn't let their unclean baby into the maternity ward... for it had been in the outside world. It was an extreme hassle, but eventually all the newborn procedures were performed, and they all went home exhausted and overwhelmed.

Salee

They had learned their lesson of choosing a location too far away that friends and family couldn't find a way to see them. Their adventure to Florida had been just that. They had a lovely home and location, but it wound up being too difficult for friends and family to make the very long trek to get to them.

Leona Valley

Leona Valley, California was their compromise. Their slice of heaven, yet still not too far away for loved ones to make the journey to see them.

Salee was a trooper, but when we went Cherry picking and she needed pain killers, we knew something was wrong.

Salee went to get her hair done and collapsed on the floor and was transported to the hospital. She had fainted, but they could not tell what was wrong with her. She had had lung surgery before... she had been a heavy smoker before meeting Vic but gave it up when they started dating.

She had an exploratory operation for constipation. Finding nothing wrong, she was released and went home.

Mookie

While in the intensive care unit, Vic was asked to bring their dog Mookie in to see her. Mookie was an English Bulldog and was incredibly well trained. Although Mookie did have a condition which brought us embarrassment on more than one occasion. During a recording of the sessions at a Bradley conference, you could hear snoring somewhere in the audience... where was that snoring coming from? Well, apparently it was Mookie! She can snore like there's no tomorrow and it sounds just like a human doing it!

Another patient in the intensive care ward gestured to Vic, bring her to me, I could use a wagging tail right about now. She was an incredible asset and made everyone smile.

Salee appreciated her coming in to see her and brighten her day. As the days passed, she was placed on hospice care waiting for the inevitable. Every day Marjie & Jay Hathaway would make the long trek out to visit with them, knowing that this couldn't go on much longer.

Over 3 weeks had passed without Salee eating or drinking a thing. They had even taken away her I.V. in the hopes of making her passing quicker and easier.

Marjie & Jay Hathaway continued to make the trip out to see them.

Salee was becoming weaker with each passing day.

Marjie & Jay walked into her room and Marjie asked, is there anything we can get for you? To their surprise and delight she asked for a baked potato! They all turned towards each other in shock and Marjie without missing a beat, instructed Jay & Vic to run up to Wendy's and get this woman a baked potato! She only had a spoon or two of the first food she had had in nearly a month! But it was the start to her recovery. She had beaten the odds and started eating and drinking and slowly was able to leave the hospital all together.

Salee was transferred to another facility and Vic felt they were not treating her well, so Vic picked her up and carried her to the car and took her to Brotman hospital.

Eventually she was released from the hospital and taken off hospice care.

This truly was a miracle and Vic & Salee joined the Hathaways for Thanksgiving dinner.

They moved from their home in Leona Valley to Marina Del Rey, to be closer to family and a hospital they liked. Salee had been getting better for a couple of years when she began to decline. They had a Condominium and were content, but Vic needed more assistance with Salee, so they moved to Culver City Retirement facility which had more accommodations for Salee's condition.

They were there for many months when Salee, again stopped eating. This time it did not seem like there would be a miracle and reverse the inevitable. Visiting often and not knowing when it might happen. We said our goodbyes and left. Vic was there and in the middle of the night, Salee drifted off into that forever sleep. Her suffering was over. Vic by her side and Mookie there too.

Transition

It was a hard transition and Vic needed some fresh air and to be near another of his true loves... the sea. He had a boat docked in the marina with a cabin and felt that he & Mookie could just make this their home. There was a place to shower and facilities just off the dock. Well, this lasted for a short time and he finally got an apartment instead.

Salee's memorial was held in the community room of Vic's apartment complex. Family, friends, and colleagues gathered to pay tribute to this pioneer.

Salee's granddaughter Kimberly was there with her new baby. Kimberly has a rare condition that she loses her voice when she gives birth. Unable to talk at the ceremony, she brought this new life to be there and complete the circle of life and show that even though there are ends... beginnings happen too!

I'm a Little Urinated!!!

Vic was a trooper! Staying steadfast during all the ups and downs of Salee's illness and passing.

Vic had moved into the apartment complex with Mookie in the hopes of settling down and being able to catch his breath and enjoy aspects of life again.

There is a saying, "if you want to make God laugh... tell him your plans!" for once again Vic's plans changed. His father had died of complications to Kidney disease. Now Vic was suffering from Kidney issues as well. He and his family agreed that this was too much for him to handle alone and he made, yet another move into a Senior Living facility in Torrance, California, (Pacific Retirement Home... now Brookdale Senior Living).

Vic got a one-bedroom apartment with a living room and made this home for himself and Mookie.

Now surrounded by others who would be there for him. They could eat together in the dining room, see performances, do artwork, watch movies, etc. He made many great and dear friends.

Vic was literally one of the youngest people living in this facility. There was a koi pond and from time to time ducks would land and have their babies around the pond and ducklings would use the pond until the wildlife team would come in and relocate the entire family to a marsh nearby. It was always fun to watch them.

Now he was settled in and had a parking place for his car... he was a catch! For he still drove! And being a doctor kinda helped too!

His condition made it so he had to get dialysis 3 times a week. A painful procedure and takes a lot out of him.

His living condition at this facility, purchased and renamed Brookdale Senior Living was home for nearly 10 years.

Vic was now not only having kidney issues, but his heart was having problems as well. At one point they

217

had to put in a stent for blood flow and redirect additional flow to his left arm. Had surgeries to splice arteries and veins together to give them locations to perform the almost every other day procedure.

He collapsed at the Senior Living facility and they rushed him to the hospital. Now they wanted to put a stent in his heart and possibly ad a pacemaker with defibrillator. For years we had seen a box on the wall of the game room at his facility with a portable defibrillator in it... now they wanted to place one on his chest.

They took Vic into the operating room and were about to start the operation when they noticed the stent that was placed in his chest already. Perplexed, the doctor told Vic that there was a chance that continuing with the operation would kill him or he could just go home... he did the latter.

Two years later things became urgent enough that they decided to try this operation again... Success! This made him feel better, stronger, and even brought his appetite back. It had been very hard to get him to eat much for months.

2018

He had arm surgery to make a new site for continuing Dialysis procedures. They thought the procedure had gone well, but it didn't. Vic's arm swelled up and he was in a lot of pain. Recovery took a long time and in so doing they transitioned him into a rehab facility.

There for a few months, he finally was able to get out of the facility. Not back to his beloved home, but to a new retirement home, Harbor Terrace Retirement Community in San Pedro, Ca. His children wanted him to be closer to them and at a facility which offered more care for him. It was a big transition! Leaving his friends and extended family behind, but he was in no shape to complain.

His new apartment is a studio setting. His children brought his creature comforts and what they thought he needed and set up everything before he ever saw the place. Downsizing is never easy, but they did a great job of making him feel at home and giving him an environment where he could be comfortable.

His new place even came with 24-hour assistance. Actually, two different women. Anna who is with him

Monday through Fridays and Dina on the weekends. Never alone, someone is there to help him both day and night.

Insights

With Blinders On...
Some of the Haze is Clearing!

I realize now, after self-examination and talks with others, that I was entrenched in a system that frowned upon anything but their teachings, methods, and/or procedures. I had and probably still have a bias against other forms of treatment and care. This includes chiropractic, acupuncture, massage therapy, holistic medicine, or anything outside of the medical box.

An Epiphany, in part, took place when I read an article about the teachings and the manipulation of women by one Dr. Joseph DeLee. He set a standard of a protocol that has literally damaged millions, possibly billions of women, their birthing care, and ultimately their babies.

It was not Delee by himself, but potentially thousands upon thousands of other doctors, hospitals, administrators, etc. that created an environment that changed the course of childbirth... possibly forever!

At the turn of the 20th century birthing began to switch from being nearly 95% at home to being nearly 95% performed in the hospitals... How on earth did this occur? And possibly more important, why?

Since the beginning of time, the only place to give birth was at home up until the creation of hospitals.

Look at the statistics that we are having today, it is abysmal. The medical standards should be revamped, and they seriously need to rethink their procedures. What they truly believe isn't helping women, and in reality is potentially doing more damage than simply letting nature run her course.

One would have to believe that the protocols that they have established were truly for the betterment of both mother & baby... At least I sincerely hope this is the case. But just like with any scientific protocol, you have to look at all sides and realize that what they have been doing is damaging the birthing environment and not helping it... in normal pregnancy & Birth.

Bias runs rampant when it comes to modern medicine. Whether it's said, taught, or inferred, doctors in general walk through life with blinders securely affixed. I can tell you this, because I am a victim and perpetuator of this stereotype.

I realized my bias when I read an article on Dr Joseph Delee. It was incredibly well written and further opened my eyes to the manipulation of the medical teachings and protocols. Delee was just one of the many who orchestrated and implemented ridiculous medical practices and routines, specifically in Obstetrics, for every birth!

What gave me an incredible epiphany was that this wonderful article, which was well written and explained what happened perfectly... was written by someone I normally would have discounted, by merely not reading the paper at all. You see the author was a person who I was basically trained to consider as a peddler of "Black Magic" or the "Voodoo" arts. I never would have read this if I had noticed first, that it was written by a chiropractor!

Bias aside, the article was right. I realized that, as a

doctor, I closed my eyes and thinking to alternative care... so much so that I still can't breakdown and see a chiropractor, acupuncturist, etc. myself! Even though I am being told that it would help me tremendously. How is taking an opioid better that getting an adjustment... perhaps I will soon find out?

Please be open minded and forgive us of our shortcomings... medicine has its place, but so does many forms of alternative care.

Be more tolerant in this world!

Shelly is a WONDERFUL Woman!!!

How does one explain exactly how Wonderful a person is and how you are grateful to them for marrying you in the first place? Having 3 incredible children with her. Raising them all to be upstanding persons who have left their own unique marks and the world is better for this!

For a time, you Shelly were the love of my life. I was so proud that you were my wife and that we conceived 3 wonderful children together. They are extended parts of each of us and I am one proud father indeed.

It is my fault that things went awry. I am incredibly sorry for hurting you by demanding a divorce. My head was not on straight, but you rose from the ashes of our marriage and stood fast at raising our children. I always supported you and our kids. Even pitching in when I could to be there for them, too. But you were left holding the bag and raising them the majority of the time... and I am incredibly thankful that you did and did one incredible job of doing this. Educated to boot... 3 Doctors, PhD, MD, & JD.

You are an incredible woman, mother, and my former wife. I hope one day you will forgive me, and I will always cherish the years we had together and our 3 legacies who have 5 extended legacies of their own, now as well.

Shelly you are WONDERFUL woman and I am forever in your debt.
Vic

My Love Affair with a Queen

After graduating from High School his folks celebrated by taking the family on an adventure of a lifetime. Traveling across the ocean blue to England and then to tour through Europe. This was usually not an option, since the resorts took up all their time during the summer months. They were between resorts and our summer was open!

This was after World War II and a chance to visit places that had survived during all of the fighting!

They got to England, France, & Italy. From the Colosseum to the Louvre... definitely sparking his sister's passion and love for the arts and their histories. So much so that she got her PhD in Art History and is currently teaching Art History at Juilliard School of Music in New York.

Now about his love affair with royalty... she was the most beautiful lady he had ever seen. So glamorous and always wearing black. She opened his eyes to love, travel and to embrace the sea. She was nearly his first true love.

He spent weeks in her embrace. Not only was she beautiful, but fierce and protected all, both day and night.

She tucked him in at night and provided sustenance throughout the days... walking with her was a thrill and brought all those who knew her incredible joy and peace of mind.

This royal figure had an average name, but was regal none-the-less... her name was Mary and she was a Queen.

Perhaps you may have surmised by now that we are talking about the great and famous Queen Mary, the one who raised anchor and straddled the ocean waves to carry them all the way across the pond to England herself. Yes, this is a ship and is now nearly visible from the balcony of his home.

She taught him great things, but perhaps the greatest is how to love & appreciate a woman and know that she is stronger than you think and is capable of incredible journeys near and far.

Words of Advice

If my time as an obstetrician is to have greater meaning, it will be by imparting some important knowledge to all those reading these words.

YOU CAN DO THIS!!!

The female body isn't broken! It has done an amazing job of birthing since the beginning of time.

PREPARATION
The issue is preparation and let me tell you here and now that no weekend class or just a few classes is going to adequately prepare you for all that pregnancy, labor, birth, and motherhood have in store for you.

BRADLEY
Best words of advice I can give any pregnant woman, "find a Bradley Teacher Today!" Nothing prepares a

woman to have better outcomes and more joyous births than ones who were prepared by utilizing Bradley techniques. The Bradley Method® is best for preparing for birth!

HUSBAND-COACH

I feel that the addition of the Husband has been an incredible and extremely valuable standard that all laboring women should have. As Dr Bradley said, *"a husband should be man enough to finish what they start!"*

"The husband or a partner can do more for the laboring woman than any amount of pain medication." I have found this statement to be accurate. Not only are Bradley Dads great, they made my job much easier. And the outcomes were typically better.

PITFALLS

Not having a high protein, balanced diet & eating a bunch of junk food!

If your medical professional hasn't recommended you taking a Bradley class... maybe you should find a different one!

AVOID

Avoid medical interventions, when not medically necessary.

Don't trust that anyone has all the answers. If you have a question... ask them! If you don't like or agree with it, get another opinion. This is your body and baby. We don't take you or your baby home with us. You ultimately live with the results. So be cautious and do your homework too!

PAIN or HARDWORK

Having a baby is painful! That being said, drugs don't eliminate all the pains or damage from surgery you might be exposed to. But Bradley classes can prepare you and potentially reduce and, in some cases, eliminate nearly all of it!

DRUGS

Drugs get to your baby! And No drug has ever been proven safe for the unborn baby. Your baby has no choice in the drugs they may be exposed to... only you can control this!

TIME

Nature gives you nine (9) months to prepare for the birth of your baby. Use this time wisely!

It takes a minimum of 3 months for your body to be conditioned with exercise. An Olympic athlete won't just take a weekend or a few weeks to prepare for a Gold medal event!

More energy is expelled during the labor and birth of a baby than a professional athlete uses during an entire game!

MAGICAL MOMENTS

Having this baby is a once in a lifetime experience. There are moments that will literally change you and bond your family together. It is an absolute shame when families do not get to experience these together. I have seen the burliest of truck drivers break down and cry at the greeting of their new bundle of joy. Please don't miss these magical moments.

HOW MANY MOMENTS ARE THERE?

Thousands upon thousands!!! Every one of them is unique, but some are more impactful than others.

NUTRITION
Eat a high protein balanced diet with 80-100 grams of protein each day.

STAY CLEAR OF...
Avoid junk foods and coffee, chocolate, processed sugars, alcohol, cigarettes, marijuana, chemicals, etc.

ALCOHOL
Are you kidding me... do not drink while pregnant!!!

MARJIJUANA & SMOKING, VAPING
Just don't! People will try and sway you and tell you how it magically is ok now... it will never ever be ok! The baby is extremely susceptible especially their brains. Neuro-apoptosis... look it up!

DOULAS
Although they can be helpful, they never should replace the husband/partner. He got you into this situation to begin with! Don't shortchange him or you. Taking Bradley classes helps train dads to not only be incredible coach's, but life partners as well. Your bonds may grow stronger and your relationship becomes more harmonious.

Doulas are there to support the couple/ family.

YOUR TEAM & PLACE
Make sure you choose doctors or midwives, and places that support the natural process.

Enjoy Your Pregnancy & Birth!

*American Academy of Pediatrics

My Kids

I must be one of the luckiest fathers alive! I have been blessed with 3 incredible biologic children and later further blessed with additional children through the marriage to my wife Salee. She had three children, Doreen, Kenneth, and Scott.

A quick rundown...

My oldest son, Ira, has a PhD and is recently retired from the Los Angeles Unified School District. Although he still does consulting for them... is this really retirement?

His wife, Evelyne has also recently retired and was a teacher of French. She is also a doctor, PhD in French Literature. Their sons Roger and Ben are doing great.

My Second son, David is a Prominent Pediatrician in Torrance, California. I rely heavily on my sons with my medical needs.

His wife Mahdu is an Allergist-Immunologist & Pediatrician. Their daughter, my grand-daughter, Diana, has graduated from Howard University with her MD. which also turns out to be my Alma mater along with her father's! Three generations of doctors graduating from Howard University Medical School in Washington, DC.

My daughter Sara is an Attorney. She travels the country setting up programs for students to excel at taking the Lawyer Bar Exam. Her two children Julia & Daniel are doing well.

Doreen was an incredible mother of two, Dawn and Kimberly.

Kenneth lives in Mammoth with his wife Karen and their son Michael.

Scott is the wild child showing up on rare occasions as he is out at sea being a long-line fisherman.

I am very proud of all my children.

With children... eventual Grandchildren are bound! At this time, I have been truly blessed with eight grandchildren.

Dawn
Kimberly
Michael
Benjamin
Diana
Roger
Daniel
 Julia

I am so proud of each of them. I wish I could express how important my family, children, grandchildren are to me.

If a man is a reflection of his seedlings that have sprouted and matured, and they too have even grown new seedlings and they too have matured... I must have done something right!

For me, my story started with the pilgrimage of both sides of my parents' families making a journey from Pinsk, Russia to the United States of America in the hopes of finding religious and social freedoms. To raise a family without limits and let them soar to new heights!

We love those who have left us and have journeyed on and hope that we have honored their dedication to family & faith.

Benjamin's Birth

My first child, Ira, was going to have a baby... with his wife Evelyne at our office across the street from Brotman Hospital. They took Bradley classes with Alice Garrido.

When labor ensued, they came to the office. Everything was proceeding normally.

After many hours, Evelyne exclaimed that she needed to go to the hospital for some pain relief.

Being that the hospital was just across the street. Vic went across the street and got a wheelchair and got her into the chair and wheeled her across the street and upstairs to the OB floor.

Settled in her room Vic checked her and found that the baby was coming soon. About 15 minutes. And medical practice dictates that it is too close to delivery to administer drugs.

The mother sustains the baby, supplying them with oxygen... once birth happens, they are on their own and life-support from mommy is no longer available.

Evelyne gave birth naturally to their first grandson, Benjamin. They were all ecstatic!

How to Work with Your Medical Team

Praise
We are incredibly lucky to be living in a time where there are tools, drugs, procedures, and especially trained personnel to aid and assist during emergency situations.

A growing number of medical personnel, facilities, and places are embracing the natural process. For this, we are incredibly thankful!

Agreement
It is very important to find people and locations which will not only permit, but highly endorse the natural process. Intervention will be kept to a minimum, unless medically necessary.

Process
The Natural process works and is best for most births.

If this were not the case... none of us would be here today.

Evidence

In Dr. Bradley's own practice, he experienced an extremely low need for interventions. With over 23,000 births... his record is very clear. "96% unmedicated Births!" with a "zero maternal mortality rate". *Husband-Coached Childbirth.* Vic also had a 0% maternal mortality rate!

Evidence & Experience

The Bradley Method® is your source for Evidence & Experience. Over the course of half a century and nearly a million births later... they boast a nearly 90% unmedicated rate.

Reassurance

We whole-heartedly believe that a woman's pregnancy team should include skilled people and facilities that can take care of extreme situations when they occur, and they do!

But just like swimming, having a lifeguard nearby is a prudent safety factor. This can be true in childbirth as well, but extreme over-responses are counterproductive. A lifeguard jumping in for a person who simply submerged their head below the water, for a few seconds... usually required no assistance.

How to Work with Your Patients

As medical professionals, we are honored guests to one of the greatest accomplishments of the human race... the perpetuation of it!

We are here to help and keep our patients safe.

Talk to Them... Not at Them!

We tend to forget that these are people who are about to have a baby that they are already responsible for. We don't take them or their babies home with us. They have legitimate questions and concerns and no matter what happens... they have to live with the consequences. So, don't be short or not thorough with them... you would want and expect the same. No, they didn't go to medical school... so what!

Don't Bring Your Own Baggage to the Party
Patients are influenced by **how** and **what** we say to them. You literally can change a situation from being positive to one needing interventions.

Leave It at the Door
Entering into a patient's room and telling them how tired they are... when it's you who are tired, can be a gamechanger.

We need to not bring down our patients. Giving birth is very hard work and the benefits from not exposing the baby to drugs is incredibly important.

Remember that drugs are poisons... poisons with benefits during medical emergencies. Normal birthing is not an emergency and we should avoid these unless absolutely necessary.

Positive Patient Responses
Assume success and give them every opportunity to achieve this.

We are Lifeguards

As medical professionals, we are here to save lives. As lifeguards, we should only jump in and save lives when medical emergencies arise.

Changing our roles from spectator to participant should only happen at points where it is truly necessary.

Thank you for reading this book about a remarkable man who became a doctor and made a real difference in the lives that he touched!

It took many years sitting down and talking to Vic to come up with this book. We hope you enjoyed it and will spread the word about The Bradley Method®

If you know, run into, or are pregnant yourself... please go to BradleyBirth.com today and find out more information that could change the course of not only your life, but especially the baby's!

Have a Happy Birth-Day!!!

James Hathaway

PREGNANT???

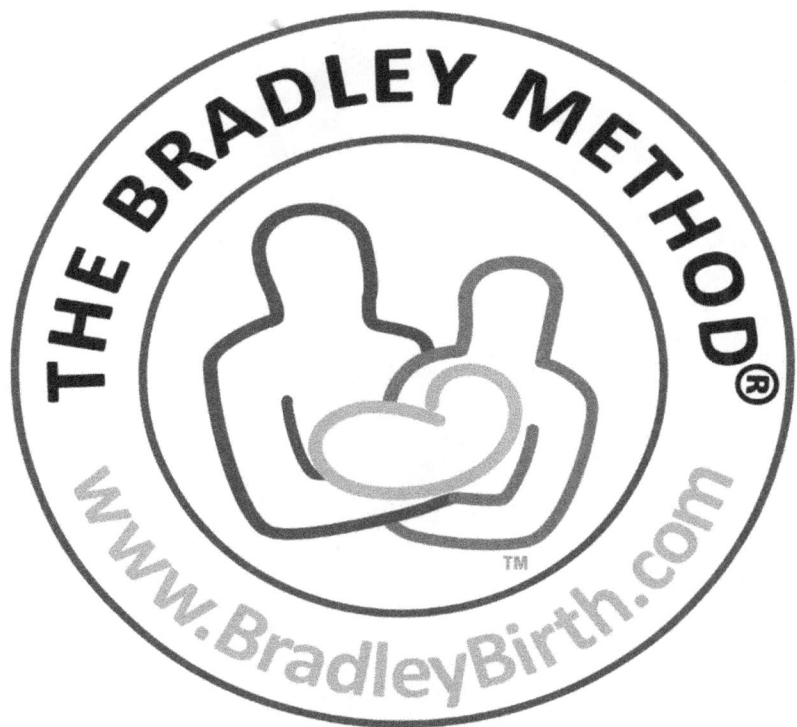

THE BRADLEY METHOD®

www.BradleyBirth.com

For Current Instructors go to:

www.BradleyBirth.com

Become a Bradley™ Teacher...
help us change the world!

 Facebook: The Bradley Method® of Natural Childbirth

Box 5224 Sherman Oaks, CA 91413-5224 (800) 4-A-BIRTH or (818) 788-6662

© AAHCC

www.ingramcontent.com/pod-product-compliance
Lightning Source LLC
Chambersburg PA
CBHW072100020426
42334CB00017B/1581